GROUPS
A guide to small group work in healthcare, management, education and research

Glyn Elwyn
Trisha Greenhalgh
and
Fraser Macfarlane

Illustrated by Siân Koppel

Radcliffe Medical Press

Radcliffe Medical Press Ltd
18 Marcham Road, Abingdon, Oxon OX14 1AA

British Library Cataloguing in Publication Data

A catalogue record for this book is available from the British Library.

ISBN 1 85775 400 X

Typeset by Advance Typesetting Ltd, Oxfordshire
Printed and bound by TJ International, Padstow, Cornwall

Contents

Preface   iv

About the authors   vii

Contributorship   ix

Acknowledgements   x

Part 1   Introduction   1
1   What is a group? And what does it do?   3
2   The group in its wider context   21

Part 2   The small group process   33
3   Setting the scene for effective small group work   35
4   Facilitation   49
5   Methods used in group work   73
6   Forming   97
7   Storming and norming   115
8   Performing   129
9   Evaluating the group process   147
10   When groups go wrong   159

Part 3   Small group work in educational settings   173
11   Evidence for the effectiveness of small group work in higher
       education   175
12   A case study of the use of small groups in postgraduate
       education: teaching evidence-based healthcare   191
13   The virtual group   201

Part 4   Small group work in organisational settings   221
14   Group problem solving and decision making   223
15   Groups across boundaries: multidisciplinary and
       multi-agency team working   243
16   Project management   257
17   Leadership   271

Part 5   Small groups in research   283
18   Focus groups   285
19   Consensus research   299

Index   311

Preface

Why another book on group work?

There is a growing body of both theoretical knowledge and practical experience which shows that small group work is an extremely powerful tool for achieving deep learning in an educational setting, building teams and effecting organisational change, undertaking complex tasks such as problem solving, strategic planning and redesigning processes. There has also been an increasing recognition of the 'group', both within sociological research and in other areas such as health, education and politics, as has been witnessed by the widespread use of focus groups, Delphi panels, and so on.

We felt that a new book on the small group process was needed for two reasons. On the one hand, many (arguably most) people in key positions in higher education and the workplace still fail to recognise the power and potential of small group work. They rely mainly or exclusively on old-fashioned, autocratic and didactic methods of teaching, training and organisational development, and they don't read the persuasive but somewhat specialist literature that supports the use of groups in a wide range of settings.

On the other hand, small group work is becoming extremely popular in many organisations. 'Away-days' are fashionable for senior management, and considered *de rigueur* by those who may have management responsibilities but little understanding of the tasks involved. Activities described variously as 'action learning', 'problem-based learning', 'focus groups' and 'learning sets' are increasingly offered to (and sometimes inflicted on) students, course participants and staff. Many people who attempt to run small groups have had no formal training and are not aware that the inappropriate and indiscriminate use of small group techniques can be ineffective, disheartening and harmful to both individuals and organisations.

Small group work methods have always been used in the world of medical education. The tradition of the 'firm' for example, where medical students are attached to a clinical team, is based on forming a small unit of peers who have the opportunity of supervised hands-on experience of talking to and examining patients to develop their clinical skills. The vocational training schemes in general practice (from the 1970s onwards) and the 'evidence-based' medicine workshops (which changed the face of medical practice in the 1990s) all use small group techniques. Many medical schools (Maastricht in the Netherlands and Newcastle in Australia, to name some well-known examples) have emulated the problem-based small group approach pioneered at McMaster,

Canada. Nevertheless, the skills of forming and facilitating small groups do not fall into place merely because organisations decide to change their learning structures. This book looks at 'groups' and their use in many spheres of life, and emphasises the need to become skilled at using them appropriately.

Who wrote this book?

This book has been written and illustrated by a multidisciplinary team of authors with backgrounds in higher education, academic research, management, organisational development, information technology and graphic design. One of us began life as a zoologist and teacher but is now a forensic psychiatrist, two are medical doctors who write and do research, and a fourth is a biochemist turned manager.

Our aims at the outset were:

1   to provide a practical guide to when and how to use small group work in educational, organisational and research settings, based on our own extensive experience of running such groups for a range of different tasks and situations
2   to encourage the wider and more appropriate use of small group work in these different settings
3   to provide an accessible summary of the theoretical principles of small group work, drawn from a range of different disciplines and specifically incorporating pedagogical, sociological and management perspectives
4   to promote the concept of the small group as a generic tool that can be used in many different environments for different purposes
5   to cross-fertilise ideas and techniques between the academic disciplines of higher education, sociological research and management, and raise awareness of common ground between these disciplines
6   to explore the application of the established principles of small group work to the virtual environment
7   to develop our own knowledge and skills in this area.

Who should read this book?

If you are getting to a position in your career, in whatever field, where you have to work in a group (or a team – hear the debate later), then you will benefit from reading this book. It will give you insights into the way that groups form, stabilise, battle and – occasionally – produce amazing results in a very short time. If you have any form of responsibility for leading (or facilitating – learn about the difference later) a group, then the book will provide a primer on how to set about the many tasks you will face. Never before has the workplace environment been changing so rapidly in either the public or the commercial sectors. One of the central theories that underpins successful change management in organisations is the need to involve, and work with, all key stakeholders both within the organisation and at the interface between organisations. The benefits of investing in the training of facilitators and applying formal principles of small group working are increasingly being recognised. The book will also provide you with examples, drawn in many cases from healthcare, of ways in which small groups are being used in education, research and management.

The book is therefore aimed at those who want to start using small group work in any of the following contexts:

*   *higher education* – this book will appeal to educators in all disciplines in higher education
*   *management within organisations* – the European Union is encouraging a new climate of industrial relations that includes support for worker participation in all decision making. NHS organisations, in common with others outside the health sector, are increasingly seeking to demonstrate their investment in, and involvement of, staff in their organisational processes
*   *research* – the focus group is a well-defined qualitative research technique which is often poorly understood and misapplied. Other techniques (nominal groups and Delphi panels) are becoming widely appreciated as useful methods of generating ideas and achieving consensus. Many of the generic skills of facilitating small groups are transferable to the setting of the research focus group.

Glyn Elwyn
Trisha Greenhalgh
Fraser Macfarlane
August 2000

About the authors

Dr Glyn Elwyn BA MRCGP MSc is a medical doctor. He gained a degree in Welsh and Drama and a medical degree from the University of Wales College of Medicine. He now works as a clinical senior lecturer in general practice, and is researching 'shared decision making' – how clinicians and patients can best share information about the pros and cons of treatment choices. He has organised many educational courses (including evidence-based healthcare workshops), and more recently has been setting up tutor-led groups to study the feasibility of using portfolios (a collection of reflections and learning experiences) as a vehicle for self-directed learning by general practitioners. Dr Elwyn also implemented a study in 1999 on the effect of asking general practices to use 'away-days' to design and implement a 'practice development plan', and is investigating the concept that organisations 'learn' and have collective memories. He is a Director of CeReS (Centre for Research Support for Primary Care) in Wales. He is the co-editor with June Smail of *Integrated Teams in Primary Care* (Radcliffe Medical Press, 1999) and he edits *Evidence-Based Patient Care* (Oxford University Press, forthcoming 2001).

Dr Trisha Greenhalgh MD, FRCP, FRCGP is a medical doctor who gained a degree in social and political sciences from Cambridge and a medical degree from Oxford. She trained as a hospital specialist (in diabetes) before moving to general practice and academic research. She is currently Director of the Unit for Evidence-Based Practice and Policy at University College London, where she provides postgraduate 'training the trainers' courses in evidence-based healthcare using small group methods. She also uses small group techniques extensively in research into the cross-cultural aspects of patient education in diabetes. Dr Greenhalgh is developing a fully web-based Master's degree course in primary care, and hopes to explore the use of small group techniques in a virtual environment. She is the author of *How to Read a Paper: The Basics of Evidence-Based Medicine* (BMJ Publications, 1997), co-editor with Dr Brian Hurwitz of *Narrative-Based Medicine: Dialogue and Discourse in Clinical Practice* (BMJ Publications, 1998) and co-author with Dr Anna Donald of *A Hands-on Guide to Implementing Evidence-Based Medicine* (Blackwell Science, 2000) and *Evidence-Based Healthcare Workbook: For Individual and Group Learning* (BMJ Publications, 1999).

Fraser Macfarlane BSc MBA MIPD is associate lecturer in health services management at the University of Surrey and an independent consultant with Granville Sansom Personnel and Management Consultancy Ltd. He was introduced to problem-based small group learning as an MBA student at the London Business School. He has since used these techniques extensively in training and team development in the work environment of health service organisations, especially NHS health authorities and trusts, and in the evaluation of a number of major projects in the academic and service sectors.

Dr Siân Koppel is a forensic psychiatrist who gained a degree in zoology at Imperial College London and a medical degree at the University of Wales College of Medicine. She completed her training in general practice before moving to forensic psychiatry. Dr Koppel is also an illustrator. Her drawings and sketches of colleagues – many of them produced during the many hours spent doodling whilst perhaps listening to eminent (and not so eminent) teachers – now grace the walls and slide trays of those who feel able to withstand the accurate caricatures represented. She has illustrated many booklets and, most recently, *Dyspraxia: A Hidden Handicap* (Souvenir Press, 1999).

Contributorship

All three authors contributed to all of the chapters, but the lead authors were as follows:

- Glyn Elwyn: Chapters 3, 4, 5, 6, 7, 8, 17 and 18
- Trisha Greenhalgh: Chapters 1, 2, 9, 11, 12, 13 and 19
- Fraser Macfarlane: Chapters 10, 14, 15 and 16.

Siân Koppel provided the illustrations and is married to Glyn.
Trisha is married to Fraser.

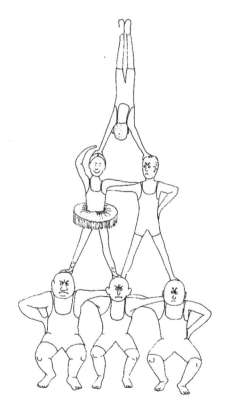

▼

Acknowledgements

We thank the following colleagues who challenged our assumptions, contributed their knowledge and guided our thinking: Lewis Elton, Anita Berlin and Simon Smail.

Mary Michel and Sharon Caple read and corrected many drafts, and the remaining errors are ours alone.

Part 1

Introduction

1

What is a group? And what does it do?

> *None of us are as smart as all of us.*
> Japanese proverb

What is a group?

There are many definitions available, and there has been considerable debate about their merits. MLJ Abercrombie, whose research into the use of small groups in higher education broke new ground in the 1960s, defined a group as *'a number of people who are in face-to-face contact, so that each of them can interact with all the others'.*[1]

Another early seminal writer on groups, Wilfred Bion, distinguished work groups from family, friendship or therapeutic groups. He defined a work group as *'a planned endeavour to develop in a group the forces that lead to a smoothly running co-operative activity'.*[2]

John Hunt, writing a decade later about group work in management, defined a group as *'any number of people who are able to interact with each other, are psychologically aware of each other, and who perceive and are perceived as being members of a team'.*[3]

Levine and Moreland define a group as several people *'who interact on a regular basis, have affective ties with one another, share a common frame of reference, and are behaviourally interdependent'.*[4]

Whatever the finer points of the definition, it is generally agreed (or at least assumed) that the members of a group have a common purpose or task, and that the interaction between them is closer, and follows a different pattern, than in casual or brief encounters. There is no fixed definition of how many members count as a group, but the dynamics of interaction change considerably if the group has more than about ten members (*see* p. 17). In practice, groups usually have between three and eight members.

The difference between a group and a team is inconsistently defined. Although Hunt and others use the terms 'group' and 'team' interchangeably, much of the recent research in social psychology has demonstrated that although teams are definitely a form of group, not all groups can be regarded as teams. For the purposes of this book, we have defined a group as a small number of people who have:

- a shared identity
- a shared frame of reference and
- shared objectives.

We have defined a team as a group in which the members distribute functions (i.e. in which there is an explicit division of labour).

We shall explore the characteristics of groups that move towards the status of a team in Chapter 8 (Performing) and in Part 4 (Small Group Work in Organisational Settings) in Chapters 14 (Decision Making and Problem Solving), 15 (Multidisciplinary Working) and 16 (Project Management).

Groups can be broadly classified into the following categories.[3]

- *Formal groups* are created as mechanisms within a wider organisation and supported by the structures and power relationships within that structure. Their functions tend to be clearly specified, their membership restricted and their control over resources limited. Formal groups include project teams and (sometimes but not always) committees, boards of directors and boards of examiners.
- *Informal groups* are looser and more erratic in their behaviour and less constrained by rules and expectations. They are usually based on friendship and/or prior shared beliefs about how things should be done. It is often in informal groups that new ideas are tested and creative solutions explored. Moreover, it is often within these informal groups and networks that real power resides within organisations, and the importance of this fact is widely recognised in the literature on social network theory.[5]

The particular focus of this book is the mechanism of the small group process (*see* Part 2) and the ways in which this process can be successfully applied in the learning situation (*see* Part 3), the workplace (*see* Part 4) and the research study (*see* Part 5).

When writing this book we were conscious that the very notion of a collection of individuals with an identity and sense of common purpose is a rare and special concept. Most so-called 'groups' would not fulfil even the most basic of the above definitions. How often, when you have been asked to lead or facilitate a group, have you been billeted into a reluctant, time-limited and somewhat confused gathering in which the members do not know (or even desire to know) each other's names, and have no shared perspective or mutual trust. Whilst we recognise that this is a common experience, this book is not about what to do when there is inadequate time or commitment to get the basics right. However, although we recoil from addressing this worst-case scenario, we also recognise that even with considerable commitment from

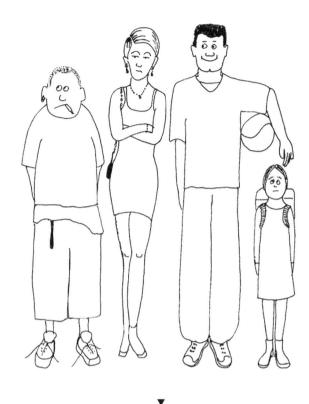

▼

Most groups are a motley crew.

the facilitator and the members, practical constraints often require compromise. The counsel of perfection suggested in some of the later chapters of this book may need to be modified in response to both external and internal reality!

What does a group do?

The *content* of group work (i.e. what the group does) varies enormously, and it obviously depends on whether the group is formal or informal, the reason why it was set up, and the task or tasks that it sets out to address. The background and context of the group are considered further in Chapter 2 (*see* p. 21).

In contrast, the *process* of group work (i.e. how the group does it) tends to follow a common pattern whatever the group has been set up to achieve. The defining features of the group process are as follows:[6]

1   *Active participation* – i.e. everyone in the group takes part in some way. Note, however, that some participants naturally have a more interactive

Table 1.1: Examples of different types of group (adapted from a number of sources)[7-12]

Type of group	Description	Recommended use
Problem-oriented learning group (see p. 17, Figure 1.1)[6]	Participants work in small groups (typically five or six members) and address complex problems chosen in advance by the tutor. They may explore any aspect of the problem that they feel is relevant. The tutor (or tutors) act as a resource for expert information as well as having a facilitator role	Arguably, this promotes deep learning through discussion and reflection. Improves motivation and encourages independent reading, literature searching and research. Is said to encourage problem-solving skills, but evidence for this is controversial (see p. 180)
Project group (see p. 257)	The group works on a joint task in four phases, namely scoping, designing, producing and presenting. The group must share ideas, identify and use individual members' skills, and take group responsibility for the range and direction of work covered. The tutor plays a supportive role	Allows in-depth study with freedom to explore different aspects of the topic and different learning methods. Requires participants to take responsibility for tutorless group work
Seminar group	Group discussion with fairly academic aims. Participants present material on a topic set by the tutor, followed by discussion and feedback. Generally, all participants prepare the material, and the tutor selects one or more of them to make a formal presentation	Promotes skills in literature searching, critical appraisal, presentation and critical discussion
Syndicate group	Participants work in tutorless groups on a structured assignment set by the tutor. The assignment generally includes a detailed set of questions or tasks with references from set books and journals. Different syndicate groups may work on different aspects of a larger problem and share their findings in a plenary session. The tutor may summarise the findings in a final lecture	Allows the tutor to exercise control over content while giving participants freedom to work without direct supervision and in their own way
Tutorial group	Participants discuss material that has been previously taught or assigned (e.g. in a lecture). They must prepare for the session and note down issues that they wish to discuss. Tutor should focus entirely on work prepared (and questions asked) by the participants	Allows participants to clarify and expand on topic material. Allows the tutor to check their level of understanding

style than others. A member may contribute actively to the group process by body language, facial expression and the sensitive use of silence, as well as by verbal expression.

2   *A specific task* – i.e. a defined and focused set of objectives. All group members must understand and agree on the objectives at the outset of the task, otherwise the group quickly becomes dysfunctional and frustrated.

3   *Reflection* – i.e. the group members incorporate experience into their shared task through an explicit process of discussion, questioning, evaluation and self-reflection.[7] Reflection is a crucial feature of deep learning (*see* p. 176).

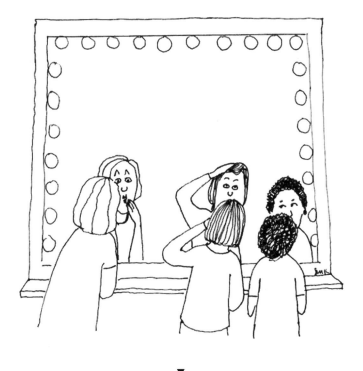

▼

Reflection is a crucial feature of deep learning.

Why is group work suddenly so popular?

Organisations of all sizes and shapes are recognising that the achievement of successful outcomes, whatever those outcomes might be, is dependent on three critical lessons learnt over some 50 years of trial and error in various fields of research and practice:[13]

- process (how something is done) affects the outcome (the results or the product)
- in general terms (but for important exceptions *see* p. 166) teams are more successful than individuals
- group member participation leads to greater commitment and success.

These principles guide a whole spectrum of activity from management (total quality management, continuous quality improvement), to education (problem-based learning, learning sets) and research methods (action research, exploration of perceptions and consensus testing). The generation of greater involvement and participation within organisations leads to an increasing use of groups and teams of all types and sizes. The tasks with which these groups or teams are charged may vary immensely – to change the ways in which 'things are done around here', to solve problems, to make decisions, to co-ordinate complex processes, to learn new skills – but all of them will face similar challenges of interpersonal communication.[14]

The rise in popularity of group work in educational settings is part of the 'liberation' approach to learning and change,[15] which is based on the premise that learning is best done by *reflecting, discussing and doing*, rather than by *receiving*. This approach also proposes that the subject matter should be of direct relevance, that participation is a necessity and that the whole person needs to be involved – their feelings as well as their intellect – so that the learning is pervasive and lasting.

This contrasts starkly with the instructivist method of learning which many of us remember from our school and undergraduate days, in which teachers typically present an external reality (a body of knowledge) which is independent of the student and which he or she is expected to assimilate. The instructivist school does not see any need to consider the impact of learning on the person and how they might integrate new understandings into their own personal contexts. Educationists are increasingly using groups to *ensure* that individuals participate actively in the learning and problem-solving tasks.

Techniques for group work

The different techniques commonly adopted for group work are summarised in Table 1.2. Note, however, that this list is neither static nor exhaustive, and that many other types of group, and uses for the techniques shown, can undoubtedly be found.

Jacques describes three broad categories of group techniques:[16]

- techniques concerned with *cognitive objectives* (knowledge, problem solving, analysis, evaluation)

Table 1.2: Examples of techniques used in group work (adapted from a number of sources)[7-12]

Method	Description	Recommended use
Brainstorming (*see* p. 91)	Should follow a three-step sequence: first, identify ideas through free discussion and record so all are visible (e.g. 'Post-it' notes, flip chart); secondly, clarify and categorise ideas; thirdly, evaluate ideas and summarise. The tutor should ensure that all ideas (however 'crazy') are welcomed and considered. The first step should continue until no new ideas are generated	Promotes initiative and lateral thinking. Good for situations in which creative solutions are required. May form the initial stage of a problem-based learning cycle
Buzz grouping (*see* p. 79)	Used in large group situations (e.g. lectures) in which an element of small group discussion is desired. Participants are asked to turn to their neighbour and discuss a topic briefly. Pairs can then be merged to form fours or sixes. The lecturer may ask for a show of hands in response to questions such as 'How many groups had someone who didn't follow the question?'	Can dramatically relieve boredom and refocus attention in a lecture. Enables the lecturer to obtain an honest estimate of misunderstandings, as the group, rather than the individual, owns the response
Controlled discussion	The tutor leads and directs discussion on a predefined topic. Participants either ask the tutor questions or (more commonly) the tutor directs questions at participants in the style of 'Socratic dialogue'	Useful for checking knowledge and understanding of presented material. Can be used with large groups, but can inhibit open discussion. If overused it may be unpopular with participants
Free discussion	Material such as a case study is circulated either in advance or at the start of the session. The tutor invites and facilitates discussion, which should range freely around the topic area. There need be no clear resolution	Encourages interaction and exploration of values and feelings. Good for controversial or sensitive material

continued overleaf

Table 1.2: Continued

Method	Description	Recommended use
Games and simulations (*see* p. 83)	The tutor introduces a game (i.e. an artificial and typically competitive situation) or a simulation (i.e. a mock-up of a work situation). The tutor explains the rules, and allocates a time period. The tutor may take part in or facilitate the exercise. The game or simulation is followed by a debriefing to clarify what has been achieved	Promotes experiential understanding and allows participants to develop skills that can be transferred to the work environment
Role play (*see* p. 81)	The participants enact a scenario, taking on various predefined roles. The tutor should first explain the background to the session and assign roles (usually as a short written brief). He or she may also take on a role. Participants then enact the scenario, which may be videotaped. Not all group members need play a role – indeed, it is better for some of them to observe. Debriefing, in which participants describe what they *felt* while playing the role, is essential for affective objectives. Participants must formally de-role before the end of the session, especially if their role was emotionally charged (e.g. that of a bereaved person)	Allows the participants to explore the feelings and perceptions of individuals in different life situations. Good for promoting communication skills
Snowballing (*see* p. 79)	The participants discuss a topic in pairs, the pairs then join to make fours, then eights, and so on. At each stage, the groups define the range of views and identify contentious aspects of the problem. Usually the tutor supplies written stimulus material (e.g. a case study) at the outset	Promotes the exchange of ideas and values, and allows participants to clarify their own views. Good for discussion of controversial or sensitive material

- techniques concerned with *creative objectives* (producing imaginative solutions, linking the emotional and the intellectual, seeing new relationships)
- techniques concerned with *social objectives* (developing individual or group awareness, developing communication skills, breaking down interpersonal barriers).

All of these techniques are covered in more detail in the chapters that follow.

Group development

In 1965, Tuckman published a seminal paper in the *Psychological Bulletin*, which argued that all groups tend to develop through four main stages, namely forming, norming, storming and performing,[17] as discussed in more detail in Chapters 6 to 8. Although Tuckman's phases are still probably the most commonly used classification for group development (and the one we shall use in this book), other taxonomies are popular in some circles. For example, Schein's four-phase sequence of dependency, conflict, cohesion and interdependence (corresponding to forming, storming, norming and conforming) is more commonly used in management.[18] As Hunt warns, these different phases should not be seen as a model to be followed, but rather as an analysis of what tends to happen.[3]

Why do people join groups?

Schein has suggested that people join groups for one of three reasons:[18]

- to achieve shared objectives (i.e. those mutually agreed by the members)
- to achieve personal objectives (i.e. those not explicitly agreed by other members)
- 'to work in a group' (i.e. to address a social need through the group process).

There is a school of thought that places unconscious motives high on the list of individuals' reasons for forming and joining groups. Bion, who is credited with being the founder of the influential group relations theory used by therapists at London's Tavistock Clinic,[19] stated that 'the human individual is a political animal who cannot find fulfilment outside a group and cannot satisfy any emotional drive without expression of its social component'.[2] He argued that for the individual, the task of establishing emotional contact with the group is a primitive and formidable act that involves both regression and loss of 'individual distinctiveness'. Indeed, Freud defined a group as 'an aggregation of individuals all in the same state of regression'![2] His theory was that large groups such as armies or churches become integrated social systems as each individual identifies (through transference) with the leader or figurehead.

Whether you are an opponent or a strong supporter of the psychoanalytical approach to relationships in groups (and between groups and the external world), you will no doubt acknowledge the powerful social and emotional dimensions of the group experience. What people *feel* when they are in a group can be as important as what they *say*, and as we shall explain further in later chapters (*see* pp. 49, 129), the skilled facilitator is able to recognise, contain and channel the emotions of the members to help them to achieve shared objectives.

What goes on in groups?

Schein described three types of behaviour that occur in groups, and which are considered further in Chapters 6 (Forming), 7 (Storming and norming), 8 (Performing) and 10 (When groups go wrong).[18]

1 *Task behaviour* is oriented to attempting to achieve the group's defined task. It includes:
    *   stating goals, defining problems, proposing how to proceed
    *   seeking and exchanging opinions or information
    *   combining, improving and building on these initial suggestions
    *   seeking or taking decisions.
2 *Group behaviour* is oriented to helping the group to survive and grow. It includes:
    *   establishing trust and mutual support
    *   encouraging appropriate contributions from all members
    *   resolving differences between members
    *   setting and enforcing standards of behaviour (e.g. about timekeeping, interrupting, and so on).
3 *Individual behaviour* is oriented to the needs and interests of the individual, and may interfere with the group process. It includes:
    *   blocking (attempting to arrest or divert the group in order to address a personal agenda)
    *   dominating other members
    *   displaying verbal or physical aggression
    *   withdrawing from the group
    *   seeking help or recognition (e.g. through self-deprecation or emotional outbursts)
    *   forming pairs or cliques
    *   grumbling or 'badmouthing' members outside the group.

These different behaviours are considered in more detail in Chapters 4 and 10.

Leading and facilitating groups

As we shall discuss in Chapters 4 and 17, leading and facilitating are very different skills, and they may be incompatible. The conventional leader of a group (e.g. teacher, tutor, coach, manager, director or 'boss') generally has a strong vested interest in obtaining a particular outcome from the group, and may be unable to tolerate dissent from his or her preferred course of action. A facilitator, on the other hand, may be deliberately chosen because he or she does *not* have a vested interest in the outcome of the group work, or a hierarchical relationship with the group members.

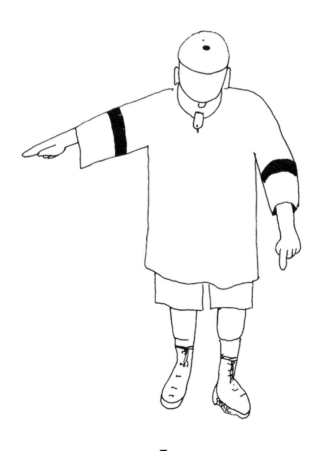

▼

Ready, steady, go!

Heron has described six categories of intervention in groups, which fall into two main groups, namely authoritative (directing, informing and confronting) and facilitative (releasing tension, eliciting and supporting),[20] which are described in more detail in Chapter 4 (*see* p. 52). Jacques divides the purpose of facilitation into the following roles.[21]

1 *The task role* involves ensuring that the group completes its task, for example by:
   - focusing members on a particular topic
   - suggesting ideas for the content of discussion
   - clarifying and elaborating the contributions of group members
   - challenging ideas and hypotheses
   - seeking or giving information
   - summarising work done so far
   - questioning the direction and depth of discussion.
2 *The group role* involves establishing and maintaining effective functioning of the group, for example by:
   - promoting a climate that is open, supportive and trusting
   - gatekeeping (i.e. ensuring that members who have a contribution to make are given the opportunity to do this)
   - managing conflict
   - relieving tension (e.g. through humour)
   - setting standards – encouraging members to establish and follow ground rules (*see* p. 102)
   - identifying and managing individual behaviours (see above) that may interfere with the group process.

As you will see from the examples given throughout this book, there is no single 'best method' for facilitating a group, or optimum balance between the more and less directive facilitation styles. The many terms used to depict leaders and facilitators (tutor, trainer, coach, teacher, facilitator, chairperson, mentor, reviewer, and so on) will give you an inkling of the subtle variation between the different roles depicted by the titles. Chapter 2 (The group in its wider context) introduces some important organisational and cultural considerations that have an important bearing on the style of leadership that will prove acceptable and effective in different situations.

In addition to the two roles described above, the facilitator of an educational group (e.g. a university tutorial) must usually strive to ensure that the learners become increasingly self-reliant, independent and confident in their studies. Groups outside the formal educational setting (e.g. learning sets) may share similar aims for the personal development of their individual members. Developing communication skills and breaking down interpersonal barriers may also be explicit aims of the group. Thus the role of the facilitator may evolve from being more authoritative to more facilitative throughout the lifetime of the group. Rather than aspiring to a single style of facilitation, we recommend that potential facilitators should aim to become comfortable with a range of styles – a challenge that is discussed further in Chapter 4.

What does the ideal group look like?

John Hunt has suggested that, for successful group work, a number of features are required.[3]

1   The members:
    • work co-operatively, not competitively
    • 'get along' with one another
    • take incentives and rewards collectively, not individually
    • are aware of the nature of the group process and the stages of group development.
2   The group:
    • has approximately five or six members
    • has autonomy to address its task
    • has an effective leader or facilitator
    • is adequately resourced in terms of time and administrative support
    • operates in the context of a supportive organisation or community.
3   The task:
    • involves all members, draws on the skills of different individuals, and requires co-ordination
    • is concrete rather than abstract
    • has a precise statement of objectives, a definite beginning and end, and measurable indicators of success.

Box 1.1 lists the determinants of group effectiveness and Box 1.2 lists the tasks and processes for which group work is particularly suited.

Does size matter?

Observational studies of naturally occurring groups with high levels of inter-action between members have demonstrated that these groups normally contain two or three individuals, and rarely include more than five or six.[22] One explanation that has been suggested is that people become confused by groups that are larger than six members, since the number of potential relationships rises sharply as each new member joins.

The number of people that any one individual can observe, communicate actively with and be involved with is around seven to eight. It is no accident that this is the typical maximum number of people usually invited to share a

---

Box 1.1:   The determinants of group effectiveness

The individual members
- Personal objectives
- Understanding of the task
- Understanding of the group process

The group
- Size
- Stage of development
- Appropriate mix of knowledge and skills
- Quality of facilitation

The task (see p. 29)
- Nature
- Salience
- Clarity
- Criteria for successful achievement

The context
- Physical environment
- Time and resources allocated
- External (organisational) factors

Box 1.2:   Types of activity for which group work is particularly suited
- Completing a complex task that requires input from multiple members (e.g. planning an induction and training programme for new employees)
- Solving problems
- Developing communication skills
- Developing and applying new ideas
- Changing attitudes of individual members
- Developing transferable skills for continuing professional education (e.g. project planning, time management, identification of one's own strengths and weakness, assumption of responsibility for learning)
- Developing transferable skills for the workplace (e.g. leadership, prioritising, mutual support)

---

communal meal with the hope of maintaining one conversation at any given time. It is impossible to control large groups for any significant period of time, and members tend to feel (correctly) that their individual influence over the group process diminishes rapidly above the threshold of five to six people.[23]

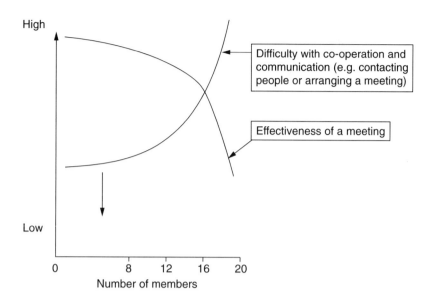

Figure 1.1:   Co-operation becomes difficult with too many members.[24]

Øvretveit described the increasing difficulty of achieving co-operation between groups of people as their number increases (*see* Figure 1.1).[24] Small group work starts to become confused when the threshold of eight or more participants is exceeded, and the task of co-ordinating a larger project team, convening a meeting or even maintaining informal contact becomes very difficult if numbers approach 15 or more members.

Some situations do allow groups to grow larger, and are usually characterised by contexts that do not require close interaction between members. In these situations the concept of group *niches* has been described. The 'niche' is the boundary that can be drawn around the group, the amount of time available for meetings, the space allocated, the resources and 'rules' about membership. If this niche has a high volume, then membership can expand, provided that there are no competing niches with overlapping interests.

As groups increase in size, they will commonly exhibit directive-type leadership, which appears to be both enabled and accepted. Perhaps this is because the group recognises that this is one of the most efficient methods of achieving co-ordination. Increasing size also leads to declining levels of participation and the development of a controlling nucleus. This can often result in declining participation and commitment, which in work environments can translate into lower levels of performance and eventually to disengagement. However, size is not the only factor that determines performance. The types of members, and whether they are similar or dissimilar, are also critical (for a discussion of diversity, *see* p. 118).

In summary, small groups that require active communication and inter-action between all members should not contain more than eight members, and ideally should have a smaller number.

Group work is not a panacea

Working in groups is becoming so fashionable that some people have started to use it uncritically in educational and research settings, or to address a host of different problems in the workplace. It is important to recognise the limitations as well as the strengths of this form of interaction. Box 1.3 lists some activities that are less suited to the small group process, and which may cause frustration if offered to a group. The impact of the nature of the task on the group process is discussed further in Chapter 2, and the specific limitations of and cautions about group work are discussed in detail elsewhere through-out this book (in particular, *see* pp. 115, 159, 175 and 221).

Box 1.3:   Types of activity for which group work is less suitable

- Simple, routine tasks that could be easily achieved by a single individual (e.g. completion of an inventory)
- Expert tasks (i.e. those requiring input largely or exclusively from an individual with unique skills or experience)
- Memorising facts (e.g. for traditional examinations)
- Individual activities (e.g. writing an essay)
- Activities involving professional intimacy (e.g. 'clerking' a patient)

References

1   Abercrombie MLJ (1979) *Aims and Techniques of Group Teaching*. Research in Higher Education Monograph No. 12 (4e). Society for Research into Higher Education, University of Surrey, Guildford.

2   Bion W (1961) *Experiences in Groups and Other Papers*. William Heinemann, London.

3   Hunt J (1992) Groups in organizations. In: *Managing People at Work* (3e). McGraw-Hill, New York.

4   Levine JM and Moreland RL (1994) Group socialization: theory and research. In: W Stroebe and M Hewstone (eds) *European Review of Social Psychology*. John Wiley & Sons, Chichester.

5   Baker WE (2000) *Achieving Success Through Social Capital*. Jossey-Bass, New York.

6   Crosby J (1997) Learning in small groups. Association for Medical Education in Europe Education Guide No. 8. *Med Teacher*. **19**: 9–16.

7   Entwhistle N, Thompson S and Tait H (1992) *Guidelines for Promoting Effective Learning in Higher Education*. Centre for Research on Learning and Instruction, Edinburgh.

8   Jacques D (1991) *Learning in Groups* (2e). Kogan Page, London, pp. 82–101.

9   Tiberius R (1999) *Small Group Teaching – A Troubleshooting Guide*. Kogan Page, London.

10   Reynolds M (1994) *Group Work in Education and Training*. Kogan Page, London.

11   Steinert Y (1993) Twelve tips for using role-plays in clinical teaching. *Med Teacher*. **15**: 283–91.

12   Saunders D, Powell T and Rolfe J (1998) *International Simulation and Gaming Research Handbook. Simulations and Games for Emergency and Crisis Management*. Vol 6. Kogan Page, London.

13   Handy C (1993) *Understanding Organisations* (4e). Penguin, Harmondsworth.

14   Handy C (1989) *The Age of Unreason*. Business Books, London.

15   Rogers A (1986) *Teaching Adults*. Open University Press, Milton Keynes.

16   Jacques D (1991) *ibid*, p. 83.

17   Tuckman B (1965) Developmental sequence in small groups. *Psychol Bull*. **54**: 229–49.

18   Schein E (1988) *Process Consultation – its Role in Organisational Development* (2e). Addison-Wesley, London.

19   French R and Vince R (eds) (1999) *Group Relations, Management and Organization*. Tavistock Publications, London.

20   Heron J (1969) *The Facilitator's Handbook*. Kogan Page, London.

21   Jacques D (1991) *ibid*, pp. 34–5.

22   Desportes JP and Lemaine JM (1988) The sizes of human groups: an analysis of their distribution. In: D Canter *et al.* (eds) *Environmental Social Psychology*. Kluwer, Dordrecht.

23   Levine JM and Moreland RL (1988) Small groups. In: *Handbook of Social Psychology*. McGraw-Hill, Boston, MA.

24   Øvretveit J (1993) *Coordinating Community Care*. Open University Press, Milton Keynes.

2

The group in its wider context

> 'What about a little light?' said Bilbo apologetically.
> 'We like the dark' said all the dwarves. 'Dark for dark business.'
> JRR Tolkein, *The Hobbit*

The importance of context

Most of this book is about what goes on *in* the group. However, people's behaviour in a group is often determined by factors that are external to the group and hence invisible or unmeasurable from within the group. The cases described in this chapter show some examples of this.

There are five important factors to consider when assessing the wider context of any group.

- Why and how have the individuals come together?
- What personal or professional 'baggage' have these individuals brought to the group?
- What is the culture of the organisation in which the group is required to operate?
- What is the nature of the task or tasks that the group is required to address?
- What external pressures does the group face?

Why and how have the individuals come together?

This question is so general that it is almost rhetorical, but it boils down to three specific aspects.

- Did the individuals choose to join the group, or were they sent?
- What attracted the individuals to sign up (or prompted someone else to sign them up)?

- What rewards or penalties (material or otherwise) will the individuals incur for attending the group?

In our experience it is crucially important for the facilitator to find answers to these questions, usually through informal means, before the group starts its business. In some groups, introductory exercises can help to determine people's reasons for attending the group and any specific constraints or influences that they face. However, such exercises should be used judiciously, as they may backfire (*see* Case 2.3, p. 24).

Case 2.1:   A reluctant group[1]

A highly experienced university tutor was commissioned to lead a session on small group teaching in a neighbouring department. He began an interactive session that he had run several times before with other groups, and which generally went down very well with teaching colleagues. After a few minutes he began to perceive hostility and lack of participation in the present group, which became steadily worse as the session continued. He called an early coffee break, and afterwards asked the delegates directly what the problem was. Their explanation was immediately forthcoming. The head of faculty had decided that small group teaching was too expensive, and they would be obliged to teach in larger groups from now on. Furthermore, several of them were shortly to be made redundant.

Case 2.2:   A hidden agenda

In a one-week intensive residential course for health professionals (*see* Chapter 12, p. 191), 100 delegates quickly settled into self-directed, multidisciplinary group work. One group leader reported that a single individual had withdrawn from the group after the first session. Even after careful reflection, none of the group could recall any incident in that session that might have alienated or distressed the absent member. The individual concerned remained resident for the full week, working alone in his room. He subsequently disclosed that he was to take an important medical postgraduate examination in 10 days' time, and he had mistakenly thought that this course was a 'crammer' for that examination.

What personal or professional 'baggage' have the individuals brought to the group?

Confident individuals may declare their personal agendas at the outset. However, less confident (or less honest) ones may conceal important goals or perspectives (*see* p. 65). Such 'hidden agendas' may include:

*   prior knowledge and skills
*   attitudes, beliefs and values
*   personality (for a further discussion of this aspect, *see* p. 73)
*   previous experience of group work (both positive and negative)
*   cultural or religious factors (this is not confined to obvious ethnic differences – for example, members of the armed forces may find it difficult to work in groups where no one is 'in charge', or where they are stripped of their conventional seniority)

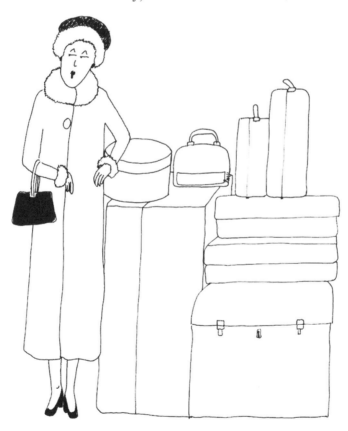

▼

Personal baggage the individual brought to the group.

Case 2.3:   Unintended social exclusion

In a teambuilding exercise, the external facilitator began by inviting all participants to state their name and say something about how they spent their
time outside work. Most people briefly described their family life and leisure
interests. One participant gave little information and was a reluctant member
of the group all day. At the end of the day, he disclosed privately to the facilitator
that, as a homosexual, he had found the 'happy families' approach to introductions alienating, and that he did not feel confident about openly sharing the
details of his private life in the group environment.

- relationships between group members outside the group (e.g. bosses or
  subordinates, individuals competing for promotion, romantic relationships)
- economic factors
- life events (recent or forthcoming).

What is the culture of the organisation in which the group is required to operate?

Broadly, social communities are either individualist or collectivist, and the
broader cultural milieu in which the group operates can influence the behaviour that goes on within the group.[2] People in individualist cultures tend to
see themselves as autonomous decision makers. Those in collectivist cultures
are much more likely to seek the views of others, and to see themselves as
interdependent; their decision-making processes will be more consultative.
Although it would seem logical for groups to be more likely to form in collectivist cultures, it seems that the opposite is true.[3] Individualist cultures have
looser arrangements and fewer fixed commitments, and so individuals belong
to a larger number of groups and more inter-group linkages are formed.
People in collectivist cultures, on the other hand, belong to fewer groups but
have stronger loyalties. Groups in collectivist cultures have been shown to
have higher levels of conformity and more clearly visible group norms.[4]

   Different work environments have different cultures. The term 'culture' in
this context encompasses the following:[5]

- the 'atmosphere' of the organisation
- the code for 'how things are done around here'
- unspoken values and assumptions that underlie how things are done
- standards used to define good or bad performance
- the ways in which individuals are recruited, trained, promoted, controlled
  and rewarded

- stories and myths about what happened to particular individuals or teams that behaved in a certain way
- organisational rituals such as journal clubs, ceremonies, social events, etc.
- subcultures and counter-cultures that exist in parallel with the 'official' version of the above.

Hunt argues that an organisation's culture is essentially determined by four variables, namely people (i.e. who works there), strategy (i.e. the organisation's broad goals and how it plans to achieve them), structure (i.e. how the organisation is made up, and what technical facilities are available) and external pressures.

Charles Handy,[6] drawing on the work of Roger Harrison, suggests that all organisations can be broadly divided into four types according to their underlying ideologies or 'cultures'.

Power culture

In this type of culture the organisation holds entrepreneurial values and is built around a charismatic leader (e.g. Microsoft, Virgin). The central (and very tangible) influence of the leader spreads through the organisation, mainly through informal communication processes. There are few binding rules, and formal group structures are rare. Control is exercised mainly by the selection and deployment of key individuals, and influence is achieved mainly through 'person power' via charismatic and informal channels.

Role culture

Most of us would call this type of culture bureaucracy and identify it with large healthcare organisations (e.g. traditional NHS hospitals and health authorities). It is characterised by a logical and visible structure, with roles and lines of accountability tightly defined by written job descriptions. Formal groups (especially committees), each with their own terms of reference, abound. Procedures for communications are explicit (e.g. by specifying who receives copies of minutes and memoranda). Performance beyond what is on the job description is not encouraged, and can be disruptive. Rules and procedures are the major method of influence, and power is achieved by position in the organisation.

Handy identifies a crucial feature of this organisation:

> *The role organisation will succeed as long as it can operate in a stable environment. When next year is like this year, so that this year's tested rules will work next year, then the outcome will be good. Where the organisation can control its environment, where the market is stable or predictable or controllable ... then rules and procedures or programmed work will be successful.*[7]

Task culture

In this type of culture the organisation, and the individuals and groups within it, are oriented towards doing a job or completing a project. The appropriate resources and the right people at the right level of the organisation are identified and then left to get on with the task. This type of organisation tends to be extremely flexible and group oriented, with groups, teams and task forces continually being formed for specific purposes and disbanded once the job is complete. Power is defined mainly in terms of knowledge or expertise relevant to the task, rewards are given on the basis of end results, and control is exercised by top management via the allocation of individuals and resources to particular tasks.

Handy suggests that 'you will find the task culture where the market is competitive, where the product life is short, and where speed of reaction is important'.[7] He cites advertising agencies and management consultancies as examples of successful task cultures. A task organisation is, at least in theory, flexible and highly responsive to change, but Handy warns that it runs into problems when money and people have to be rationed, whereupon individuals become demoralised, teams within the organisation are forced to compete for resources, and top managers find themselves imposing control via old-fashioned means. In short, the task culture is inherently unstable and tends to change to a role or power culture where resources are limited.

Person culture

Here the organisation itself is barely visible, and exists only to serve the individuals within it (e.g. barristers' chambers, architects' partnerships and hippy communes). The individual sees the organisation as no more than a place to 'do their thing'. Influence is shared, and its power base is defined by expertise. Few organisations succeed in making this their dominant ideology, but it is common for individuals within an organisation (and within a group) to adhere strongly to the person culture. The old-fashioned university professor, the idiosyncratic consultant surgeon and the eccentric schoolteacher are all stereotyped examples of person-oriented individuals operating within a role culture – and Handy warns that they can be extremely difficult to manage.

Summary

In general, an increase in size pushes the organisation towards a role culture, although radical decentralisation and careful strategic planning may allow size to increase without an excessive increase in bureaucracy. Rapidly changing technologies require a task or power culture, but routine and 'programmable' tasks may be better suited to a role culture. Role cultures are also beneficial where there are clear economies of scale (e.g. from investment in an expensive piece of equipment, or use of the limited expertise of one individual). An organisation whose goals are expressed in terms of quality standards for a product or service is well suited to a role culture, as monitoring and account-ability are readily implemented, at least in theory. Goals that are expressed in terms of economic growth are best served by a power or task culture.

People with a strong need for structure, security and predictability will be more comfortable in a role culture, while those with a strong need for individuality and creativity will prefer a task culture, and those with a need to establish their identity may seek a power culture. In general, task cultures require high input in terms of human resources (Handy's 'resourceful humans' – clever, creative, self-motivated and with strong interpersonal skills).

Groups that work within an organisation (e.g. a company or university) can be affected by the success or otherwise of their parent institution. Organ-isations in decline often generate inter-group rivalries for resources, and generate a climate of spiralling protectiveness and limited communication between departments.[8] Each group will tend to try to control its fate by engag-ing in a variety of political activities, and we need to be aware of the roles that usually emerge in such situations. Levine describes the 'scout' who goes out to bring in information and resources, the 'ambassador' who provides the export function, and the 'sentry' who controls these processes.[9]

Case 2.4:   Group decisions in a person culture

A seven-partner GP practice in a large health centre went through an acrimonious split and subsequently consisted of five different practices (three single-handed and two small partnerships) under one roof. Each practice became steadily more individualised over the years. Nursing and ancillary staff were shared, and had to develop different ways of working to meet the diverse requirements of the different doctors. Various 'guidelines' could be found pinned to the wall in the treatment room and the secretaries' office, listing how each doctor pre-ferred things to be done.

Even after the split, the doctors continued to meet together on a monthly basis for 'administrative' purposes. Decision making in the group was extremely difficult, and this was attributed to the personal animosity between various ex-partners. However, as the years went by and retiring individuals were replaced by new partners, decision making failed to improve even though all of the doctors now got on very well with each other on a personal level. Suggestions made by any one member would typically be blocked by one of the others on the grounds that 'I can't see how this is going to help *my* practice'. The problem was that the organisation had developed a strong person culture, and the individuals within it found it difficult to consider group objectives even when it was in their long-term interests to do so.

In addition to issues of organisational culture, groups frequently have to deal with different social, religious and professional cultures among the individual members (for a more detailed discussion of this topic, *see* Chapter 15, p. 251).

What is the nature of the task or tasks that the group is required to address?

As we indicated at the end of Chapter 1, some tasks are more suitable for group work than others. Not only are some tasks better done by individuals, but the nature of the task can profoundly influence the group process itself. Steiner has produced a set of five questions about a task that allow predictions to be made about the likely success of the group in achieving it.[10]

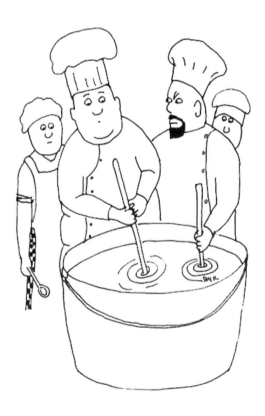

▼

Some tasks are done better by individuals.

Is the task divisible?

Tasks may be either:

- *divisible* – i.e. they can be broken down into subcomponents (e.g. organising a surprise birthday party, launching a boat, or planting an allotment) or
- *unitary* – i.e. indivisible (e.g. marking an essay, adding up a sheet of figures).

Large divisible tasks may be broken down into smaller ones until the components are themselves indivisible. In the birthday party example, these components might consist of organising the venue, booking the band, making the decorations, buying the food and drinks and making the cake. Although the last task might reasonably be divided into baking and icing the cake, there is arguably little sense in dividing these subcomponents any further.

Is the focus on quantity (of output) or quality (of performance)?

Tasks may be predominantly:

- *maximising* tasks, which entail doing as *much as possible* of something or
- *optimising* tasks, which entail doing something *as well as possible*.

The tug-of-war is the prototypical 'maximising' group task. It does not matter too much about the positioning of everyone's feet or the utterance of expletives – the objective is to exert as large a force as possible on the rope. In contrast, brain surgery (an 'optimising' task) requires maximum attention to precision, accuracy and other aspects of quality performance, rather than on the number of operations completed per unit time!

How are individual inputs related to the group's performance?

The inputs of individual members to the group process may be:

- *additive* – individual inputs are simply added together (e.g. pulling on a rope, digging a hole)
- *disjunctive* – the group selects the 'best' of the individuals' contributions (e.g. answering a quiz question, selecting the best of a range of options)
- *compensatory* – the group produces an approximate average of individuals' contributions (e.g. estimating the exact time of day when no one has a watch)
- *conjunctive* – all group members must contribute to the product (e.g. playing a football match)
- *discretionary* – the group purposefully decides how individual inputs will contribute to the group product (e.g. the group decides to vote on the

answer to a sports quiz, or alternatively it decides to allow the most 'sporty' person's answer to count).

How are group members interdependent in terms of their outcomes?

The individual members of a group may each either gain or lose from the group's product. Overall, the relationships within the group may be:

- *co-operative* – where there is commonality of interest and everyone is likely to gain from working together (e.g. playing a 'friendly' football match, putting on a show)
- *competitive* – where there is conflict of interest, often where group members are rewarded individually and scored against one another for an aspect of the group process (e.g. when students are graded individually according to what they say in a group seminar – an inadvisable assessment mechanism which invariably leads to attempts to 'score points' off one another) or
- *mixed* – where the group members are not in direct competition but have something to gain from pursuing individual goals (e.g. a premier league football match in which the players are being watched by the selectors of the national team).

The question of whether individual or group work is 'best' for a particular task is not straightforward, but it is influenced by the answers to these questions. For example, an additive, maximising task such as a tug-of-war clearly requires all hands on deck. The group's output will be the sum of the individuals' outputs (if, and only if, there is no 'loafing').[10] In contrast, an indivisible, disjunctive task such as giving the right answer to a quiz question requires at least one individual to have the necessary knowledge or expertise, but there is little additional gain if several people can supply the same input. In this case, the group's performance is equal to that of its most competent member. Finally, a divisible, conjunctive task such as playing a football match or abseiling down a precarious cliff requires everyone's input. Often the group's success will be determined by the input of the least competent member. The question 'Are many heads better than one?' is considered further in Chapter 14, p. 231.

Case 2.5:   A competitive task

The four short-listed applicants for a senior pharmaceutical executive post are invited to a 'trial by sherry' reception followed by a group task, which is observed through a one-way mirror by the appointments committee. The applicants are asked to work together to design a possible restructuring of the geographical regions in which the company's sales representatives work, from five regions (the present arrangement) to three.

continued opposite

All of the applicants quickly engage with the task, and there is rapid discussion in which everyone submits suggestions. Each suggestion is articulate and well reasoned. However, after 20 minutes the group has still not listed or prioritised potential solutions, and the discussion has degenerated into polite but unproductive small talk.

It is clear to the unseen observers that the individuals in the group are concerned only with putting their own suggestion on record, and in making sure that no one else's suggestion takes priority over theirs. Consequently, the group's objective has been overlooked.

What external pressures does the group face?

It is easy when working in a group to forget that people and organisations outside the group have a strong vested interest in what goes on. They frequently control resources and can often call the tune even though no one in the group itself shares their perspective. In Chapter 15 (Groups across boundaries) we shall explore the potential problems of competing loyalties in relation to inter-agency and multidisciplinary groups. In Chapter 16 (Project management) we shall discuss the importance of stakeholders in influencing the group task and its productivity (in particular, *see* pp. 267 to 269).

Conclusion

When groups or teams come together, they inevitably do so in a wider social, cultural and organisational context. When groups 'go right', this is often not only because the right group processes are occurring (*see* Chapter 8), but also because the right people have come together for the right reasons to address an appropriate task, and they have the right support from the right external stakeholders. Conversely, when groups go wrong (*see* Chapter 10), it may not simply be the group process that is failing. Perhaps, given the wider context and the nature of the task, the group should not have been formed at all.

Case 2.6:   Pressure from outside

A college of further education seeks to develop a programme of distance learning that runs across all faculties and draws students from beyond the immediate catchment area. A working group is appointed whose remit is to produce specific recommendations and a business plan before a forthcoming meeting of the college's executive. The group quickly identifies that a market research exercise is needed to identify the subject areas in which a potential overseas market exists. They plan this exercise and allocate tasks, but quickly realise that the work will not be completed before the executive meeting. The group is divided about what to do next – refuse to meet the deadline or produce a business plan based on unreliable estimates of demand.

References

1   Tiberius R (1999) *Small Group Teaching – a Troubleshooting Guide*. Kogan Page, London.

2   Triandis HC (1989) The self and social behaviour in differing cultural contexts. *Psychol Rev.* **96**: 506–20.

3   Curtis JE, Grabb EG and Baer DE (1992) Voluntary association in fifteen countries: a comparative analysis. *Am Soc Rev.* **57**: 139–50.

4   Bond R and Smith PB (1996) Culture and conformity: a meta-analysis of studies using Asch's line judgement task. *Psychol Bull.* **119**: 111–37.

5   Hunt J (1992) *Managing People at Work* (3e). McGraw-Hill, London.

6   Handy C (1993) *Understanding Organisations* (4e). Penguin, Harmondsworth.

7   Handy C (1993) *ibid*, p. 186.

8   Krantz J (1995) Group process under conditions of organizational decline. *J Appl Behav Sci.* **21**: 1–17.

9   Levine JM and Moreland RL (1998) Small groups. In: *Handbook of Social Psychology*. McGraw-Hill, Boston, MA.

10   Steiner ID (1972) *Group Processes and Productivity*. Academic Press, New York.

Part 2

The small group process

3

Setting the scene for effective small group work

> *Tell me the landscape in which you live and I will tell you who you are.*
> José Ortega y Gassett (1883–1956)

The importance of the physical environment

Ortega y Gasset, the Spanish philosopher, believed that life consisted of an intense dialogue between oneself and one's environment. Winston Churchill was similarly aware of the power of architecture and said, 'we shape our buildings, and afterwards our buildings shape us'. Although the choice of settings available for small group work may well be limited, it is clearly important not to dismiss the effect that a building or room has on the way in which people interact.

> *The way we perceive a place is not just a visual experience. The form of the building is important, but the textures, smells and sounds play an equal or greater role. The combination of these sensory experiences – the way wood feels to the touch and the resonance of our footsteps as we walk across the polished timber floor – are a major part of our reading of a place.*[1]

Christopher Day, considering the effects that buildings have on human interaction, pointed out that, 'other than architects, few people think about architecture, but many people feel it'.[2] We spend most of our time in buildings of one type or another, and pay little attention to the effect they have on our lives. As an illustration of the effects of environment on groups, imagine a group discussing the ethics of euthanasia in a bar-lounge of a rather tacky hotel. Compare the effect of holding the same discussion in the minimalist décor of a prestigious research institution. The structures in which we are enveloped and the physical and emotional journeys that we have to make to enter them largely determine the way in which we talk to one another, albeit unconsciously perhaps. A meeting of people seated in armchairs around a log fire may achieve a convivial atmosphere, but would do little to encourage a rational approach to tough decisions required in a dysfunctional organisation. On the other hand, the impersonal environment of the typical institutional seminar room might provide the right level of institutional anonymity to help a group of strangers start getting to know one another.

There is a specialised literature which discusses the relationship between environment and behaviour,[3] which is a theme that has been traced back to the attempts of animal behaviourists in Europe to 'design a better cage' for captive wild animals in zoos in the 1940s in Europe (Julienne Hanson, personal communication, University College London). David Canter has studied the way in which different types of interior, such as flat or sloping ceilings, provoke different responses in people.[4] The study of these interactions is known as environmental psychology – a field in which buildings have been described as our third 'skins'. The first skin is our real skin, the second consists of our clothes, and the third skin consists of the structures that enclose us, however they may be constructed. It was in the early 1950s that Kurt Lewin drew attention to the interaction between individuals and their immediate environment and suggested that behaviour (B) is determined by a combination of personality (P) and environment (E). Hence the familiar equation B = *function* (P × E).[5] By the 1970s, there were researchers who called themselves environmental psychologists studying environmental contexts and consequent behaviour.

The research themes in this field indicate the importance of considering the impact that a particular setting will have on the group dynamic.[6]

Attention

Understanding human behaviour starts with understanding how people notice their environment, both consciously and unconsciously.

Perception and cognitive maps

Information about buildings and spaces is stored in the brain as spatial networks known as *cognitive maps*. These structures link an individual's recall of experiences with their perception of present events, ideas and emotions, and will influence how they work together with others and carry out any plans.

Preferred environments

People tend to seek out places where they feel competent and confident, and where they can make sense of their environment while also being engaged with it. Research has expanded the notion of preference to include *coherence* (a sense that things fit together) and *legibility* (in the sense that 'illegible' means one can get lost easily!). For people to enjoy working in an environment, it should have enough complexity and mystery to make it worth learning about. Preserving, restoring and creating a preferred environment is thought to increase people's sense of well-being and their behavioural effectiveness.

Environmental stress and coping

Noise and temperature are well-recognised stressors, but there can be other less obvious environmental problems, such as inappropriately scaled settings or personal territories where the flow of information or stimuli cannot be managed.

When groups become firmly established, they often start to adapt their environment, mark it out as their own and defend the territory against outsiders.[7] It is important to be aware of these issues, particularly as a potential newcomer or facilitator. Territory serves many purposes – it establishes privacy and social identity, and protects resources for exclusive use by group members. This can be immediately identified in many organisations when departments within the same parent company or university vie for attention and rewards. Groups can also apportion spaces by virtue of status or seniority, and eventually spaces become interpreted in special ways, so that the group feels that the space is a necessary determinant of success.[8] The group has become 'space dependent'. Threats to move, change the structure or allow other uses will generate a strong sense of protection among group members.[9]

Choosing the venue: home or away?

Apart from influencing decisions about clothing (selecting the correct 'camouflage' to wear at conferences in swanky hotels or for encounter group weekends in the country can be tricky), the venue will also largely determine the prevailing mood of the group. The context and its associations inevitably shape the level of formality and the attitudes to working or learning that emerge. For example, trying to hold a business partnership meeting in one partner's own home or physical space usually results in territorial biases and a reluctance to challenge the host's views.

Identifying and trying to resolve organisational problems by holding meetings at the workplace is often extremely difficult. Tackling management problems such as team dynamics, forward planning, process redesign and strategy requires open communication methods that are difficult to achieve in the existing workplace because individuals are constrained by their existing

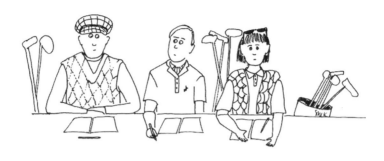

▼

Adopting the correct camouflage.

patterns of behaviours. Hierarchical relationships are reinforced by established seating patterns. Opportunities to generate new insights and challenge unproductive practices need a 'distancing' effect.

For these reasons, many organisations and teams find that it is better to move to a neutral environment for a creative group experience. A novel setting helps to break down the territorial stances of senior members, and on a practical level it avoids the potential interruptions and distractions which inevitably occur in work settings. Planners of small group work should give these issues considerable attention, particularly if the small group is charged with the task of solving problems, learning new skills or providing new ideas. However, just because a commercial venue offers 'awayday' facilities this does not mean that it is right for your event. Mundane problems such as traffic jams *en route* or lack of car-parking facilities can get the entire team off to a bad (not to mention late) start.

Why is it that some spaces seem to have the effect of inducing conversation, whilst others instil a sense of calm and reflection? The impact of light, ventilation, the resonance of the walls and other fixtures all play a part. Day has pointed out that there are 'shapes like round tables, which bring people into community, and others like uninterrupted corridors or long rooms, which do not'.[2] Some buildings, such as the Guggenheim Museum in Bilbao with its sweeping curves reminiscent of an upside down, ocean-going liner clad in titanium scales, challenge the conventional ways in which spaces are designed. You may have buildings in your area that are unusual in some way, yet which could accommodate at least some of your group work processes. Whatever setting you choose, try to match the environment to the underlying goals of the group.

Research projects use small groups in very specific ways and must avoid (and be seen to avoid) the potential influence of the setting on the interview or interaction. For instance, a researcher who is interested in using focus groups to study the factors that influence patients' satisfaction with a healthcare service should avoid using healthcare settings (such as hospitals or GP surgeries) for the interviews, even though such buildings may come cost-free and contain an accessible and convenient sample of informants! Ensuring neutral venues is as important as employing facilitators who are not paid-up members of the healthcare service you are trying to evaluate!

Attention to comfort: Maslow's hierarchy of needs

The performance of individuals in small groups is particularly dependent on their perception of comfort, both with the other people present and with their surroundings. It can be argued that the behaviour of individuals at a particular moment is usually determined by their strongest needs. Abraham Maslow developed an interesting framework that helps to explain the strength of certain needs. His 'hierarchy of needs' model categorised human needs into five levels (*see* Figures 3.1 and 3.2).[10]

You would be foolish to ignore your group members' basic need for regular food and drink. The quality and timing of the tea and coffee provided is

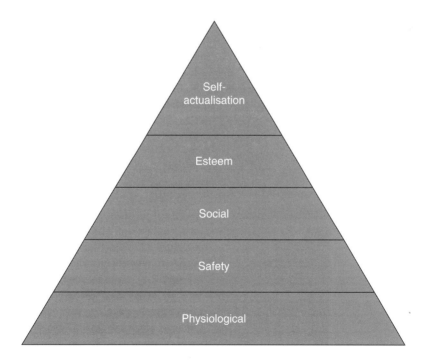

Figure 3.1:   Maslow's hierarchy of needs.

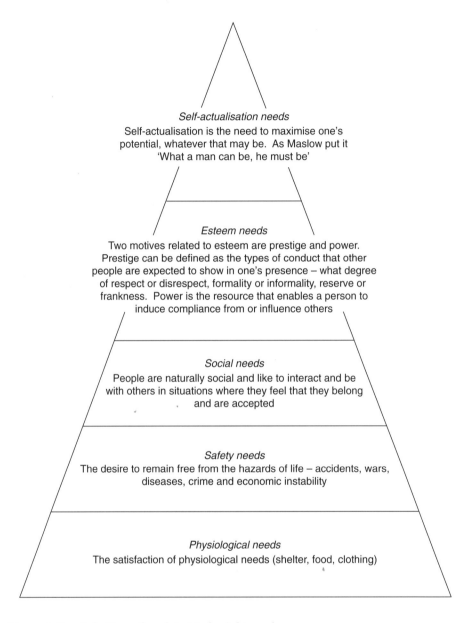

Figure 3.2:   Definitions of needs in Maslow's hierarchy.

surprisingly often rated the 'worst feature' of the entire event. Make sure that you cater for special tastes and diets (e.g. by offering herbal tea, water or soft drinks as alternatives).

Environmental factors such as light and heat can also affect group performance, and are especially important in the more mundane settings of office and factory environments. It is often not possible to modify the arrangements for light or heat, but be proactive with curtains, blinds and window-catches to ensure that the sun's glare is avoided and that temperatures are comfortable.

As far as is feasible, check beforehand about the possibility of intrusion by noise. Many group sessions have been interrupted by building work or have collapsed into unruliness as a result of constant disturbance by other activities. Mobile phones are a particular nuisance, and if you have sufficient administrative back-up, you may consider running a 'cybercrèche'. Take a cardboard box about twice the size of a shoebox and divide it internally using corrugated cardboard into a dozen or so segments, each of which holds a mobile phone (or bleeper). Prepare some A5 slips of paper giving the name of the owner of the phone, which room they will be in, and any specific messages they may be expecting.

At the beginning of your meeting, announce that mobile phones should either be turned off or left in the cybercrèche (which you should hold up for the group to view). Delegates should fill in an information form and wrap it around their phone, securing it with a rubber band. During the group work, your administrator should guard the box and answer any calls with the response, 'He/she is in a meeting right now, and will be collecting messages at ... o'clock. Shall I get him/her to ring you back then?'

Information that should be given to participants before the group meets

If possible, let your participants have detailed information about your venue and an idea of the range of activities before the group meets. This can help to reduce levels of anxiety and inform decisions about the type of clothing to be worn (e.g. short skirts should be avoided for some exercises and seating arrangements).

Seats and seating

The ideal setting allows a high degree of flexibility so that groups of different size can be formed as the need arises. On longer courses, personal time and quiet space for individual work are required, as well as the ability to convene as a large group in a location where good-quality audio-visual aids are available.

Small groups tend to work together for at least a couple of hours at each session (usually a minimum of one hour). Seating should therefore be as comfortable as possible, and it is worth expending some effort at the outset to get it right. Many traditional teachers have difficulty with the concept of moving or changing the furniture, but it is vital if small group dynamics are to function effectively.

Note the thresholds for the distances which people consider comfortable within groups. Hall noted that the upper range for talking in a casual voice is about 8 feet (slightly more than 2 metres) and that with normal vision facial expressions can be recognised at 12 feet.[11] It could be argued that it is these physical dimensions which limit the functional size of small groups, and not the number of possible interactions. Alexander's classic text points to a general truth, which facilitators will recognise:

> ... a small group discussion will function best if the members of the group are arranged in a rough circle, with a maximum diameter of about 8 feet. At this diameter, the circumference of the circle will be 25 feet. Since people require about 27 inches each for their seats, there can be no more than about 12 people round the circle.[12]

Chairs should ideally be movable so that subgroups can be formed as necessary, either into different formations of a full group, or into smaller subsets (e.g. pairs or threesomes, etc.) (*see* p. 79). Chairs should also be of equal 'status' and comfort. It is unwise to have a few hardback wooden chairs mixed in with either low armchairs or office chairs on castors. The variable heights and inevitable jostling for the best seats will undermine the equanimity of the group dynamic.

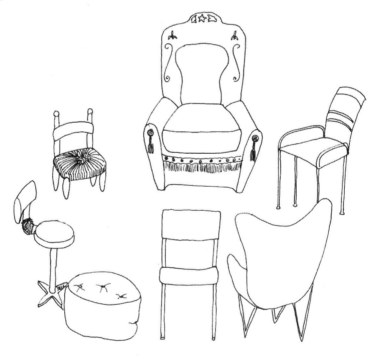

▼

Chairs should be of equal 'status' and comfort.

Some facilitators insist that small groups sit without desks or tables so that individuals are fully aware of each other's body language. The usefulness (or not) of sitting around a table depends on the nature of the learning task. In general, a table may exclude some body language from view and encourage reticence. However, insisting on a furniture-free format can be cumbersome, especially if the group needs to work together to consider written material. Sitting around a set of small tables is a perfectly feasible alternative, provided that attention has been given to the forming process (*see* Chapter 6).

The typical small group format is a circle in which all of the group members can see one another. This arrangement encourages maximum participation and allows all members to gauge each other's turn-taking strategies. However, if the group number exceeds ten it can be difficult to achieve cohesion without forming subgroups. The number of possible contributions to a point or issue and the potential for conflicting viewpoints means that a large group will always contain unvoiced comments and opinions that will influence the group dynamic.

Another common arrangement is the horseshoe. This introduces a degree of hierarchy, thereby clarifying the role of the facilitator and increasing his or her control over contributions made by members. Most facilitators try to modify large groups into smaller task groups and then facilitate by moving between units that are working in closer alliance.

Other formats are possible, such as the cabaret and boardroom style, but the fragmentation of the former and the formality of the latter – if they are the only seating arrangements used – will militate against small group processes being undertaken in any real depth.

Chairs arranged in rows emphasise the position of the individual who faces the group, and suggest an instructor role for the facilitator, which may be at odds with the adult learning approach espoused by the small group ethos.[13]

A very large room (such as a dining-room or a meeting-room) provides an opportunity for group members to determine or change the 'shape' of the group by rearranging the chairs. Group members may adjust the spaces so that some members are excluded. Others may exclude themselves by dropping out of the circle, or by adjusting the spaces between chairs to create unequal subgroupings. The facilitator should be aware of the danger of members manipulating space in this way, and if necessary they should intervene. These details may seem unimportant, but the power of spatial language should not be underestimated.[14,15]

Very often we have little control over the seating arrangements and are required to conduct group work in the most unsuitable of settings. It may be possible to overcome many problems, and some examples are suggested below.

* If at all possible, visit the room beforehand. If difficulties are likely, raise the issue in the ground rules and ask members to be aware of inter-member

spatial arrangements. Highlighting the problem in this way legitimises your intervention if you subsequently ask members to modify their positions.

- If you find yourself in a venue that has bland, institutional-type interiors where everyone gazes wistfully out of the windows at beautiful lawns, consider asking whether the group would like to move outside, perhaps to meet in the shade of a tree. (Note that administrators can become perplexed when they see flipcharts being uprooted, but this anxiety can usually be assuaged with promises of safe retrieval.)
- Offer the group members a short break from the restrictive seating plan by asking them to form pairs or triads who are asked to go for a short walk or take an early coffee break to discuss a task. This can be an alternative to the previous option, even in winter!
- Break the 'imaginary' rules. If you are stuck with a classroom that has lines of fixed desking, ask the group members to sit on the desks facing one another.
- Reconvene your group into smaller groups around two flipcharts. This will give you an insight into the way in which the group has designated the role of reporter and scribe, and whether one member has assumed both roles.
- If you find that your venue is totally unsuitable, ask the group to help you to consider some radical alternatives. Explore all of the potential spaces (e.g. entrance halls, corridors) or even consider decamping to a restaurant.

Resources

The essential components of a facilitator's kit are easily transportable.[16,17] Apart from the flipchart paper and stand (which are normally provided in a hired venue – but check well in advance just in case), most facilitators ensure that they take the following equipment with them wherever they work.

Adhesive (Blu-Tack®)

This is an essential item (provided that its use is allowed) which enables almost any vertical surface to be used as a form of display. It works well as a facilitator's 'worry ball' when times are difficult, and as a means of securing paper or other items to available surfaces when groups are working well. Do remember to check whether Blu-Tack® can be used on walls, as some surfaces can be damaged by it.

'Post-it' notes

An assortment of movable notes can be used in many ways. The large size (approximately A5) is particularly useful for collecting ideas during brainstorming or nominal group work (*see* Chapters 5 and 18). It avoids the rather cumbersome task of writing every suggestion on a flipchart, and it overcomes the tendency to comment on or qualify contributions before being invited to do so. The ability to move and regroup these items adds immensely to the collaborative mood that is generated during a good brainstorming session.

Thick-tipped pens

It is best to use the water-based (non-bleeding) variety for flipchart work. Bring a plentiful supply of these in a variety of colours. You should carry one per group member so that each member can work independently if necessary.

Clock and timer

When groups start working well together, it is amazing how time seems to fly by. On the other hand, tedious group work can result in furtive glances at wrist-watches and neck-twisting attempts to check the wall-clock. Strict timekeeping is an essential feature of good facilitation, and the warm 'fuzzy' nature of group work is no excuse for a lackadaisical attitude to starting and finishing sessions. One way of making this completely explicit is to have a physical reminder available. An excellent method is to set time limits for each piece of work and to designate one member to time-keep (or alternatively to set an alarm) accordingly. Group members soon realise that time is a crucial resource when there are many individuals who want 'air-time', and should learn to respect the need to plan its use accordingly.

Flipchart paper

Many facilitators like to have two flipchart stands available so that lists and diagrams can be compared and developed. Some organisations have invested in electronic whiteboards with automatic links to printers or photocopiers. These can provide almost spontaneous access to every individual of the combined deliberations of the group as captured on the whiteboard. However, the advantage of flipcharts is the way they can be moved around to occupy new positions, or into smaller group arrangements, and therefore integrated into the group process. This interaction with a blank sheet of paper at close proximity seems to provide an intimate means of individual and group expression which is difficult to achieve in the way that most electronic whiteboards are set up.

Audio-visual equipment

Small group facilitators are right to be wary of overhead, slide or video projectors. Of course, this type of equipment is essential when presentations are being conducted, and should then be used to its maximum potential. However, small groups are not opportunities to provide 'lectures' to a small number of people, and there is a good argument for removing this type of equipment until it has been agreed that a more formal presentation is required. One of the more irritating group experiences is to watch valuable time pass by while a nervous presenter is attempting to fix a technical problem with an overhead projector or (worse) 'state-of-the-art' computer or video, when all that the presentation in fact requires is a quick sketch of ideas and concepts for wider debate.

Optional extras

The list of potentially useful equipment for group work is endless. Some authors suggest having items such as scissors, paper clips, rubber bands available – and a box of tissues handy in case role plays become highly charged (*see* Chapter 5).[18,19]

Using flipcharts

Flipcharts are essential and they are also great fun to use. Charts can be used without tripods, although it is well worth having two stands if they are available. If you do decide to break the 'rules' listed below, at least make sure that you are aware of them, and ask the group's permission to do so.

* Stand to the side as you write, in order to avoid turning your back to the group.
* Write in a large legible hand that is visible to the whole group.
* Use thick bold colours (avoid yellow and pink).
* Hold three pens between the fingers of your spare hand to avoid having to search for a pen of a particular colour.
* Use colour to make logical rather than arbitrary distinctions (three colours are ample).
* When you are recording suggestions, use the contributor's exact words if possible – avoid paraphrasing without permission.
* If you have asked for contributions, accept them – beware of acting as a censor.

Experienced facilitators (*see* Chapter 4) will avoid overusing flipcharts, as to do so reinforces hierarchy and reduces group autonomy. Note that there is a point within small groups when one or more individuals will seek to take control, usually demonstrated by a concerted move towards the flipchart, often while brandishing an open marker, and this situation needs to be handled carefully.

Flipchart use during 'brainstorms' requires a different approach to the summarisation of a long discussion. It can often be extremely useful to ask one or more members of the group to join in the writing activity so that every suggestion is caught as the 'storm' breaks out (for more details on brainstorming, *see* Chapter 5, pp. 91 to 93). When a chart is used as a means of concluding a debate, for instance, avoid rushing to put pen to paper. There is a great temptation to get the words down, yet by their very existence they may freeze what was previously a fluid creative exercise as the group worked towards an agreed definition or statement. A tentative approach works well in this situation. Distribute flipchart paper and pens so that pairs or triads can work on their thoughts, and allow discussion so that agreed good ideas or phrases will make it to a 'summary' chart in due course (for a discussion of snowball techniques, *see* Chapter 5, p. 91).

References

1   French H (1998) *Architecture*. Simon and Schuster, London.

2   Day C (1999) *Places of the Soul: Architecture and Environmental Design as a Healing Art*. HarperCollins, London.

3   Sommers R (1969) *Personal Space: the Behavioural Basis of Design*. Prentice Hall, New York.

4   Canter D (1996) *Psychology in Action*. Dartmouth, Aldershot.

5   Lewin K (1952) *Field Theory in Social Science*. Tavistock, London.

6   De Young R (1999) Environmental psychology. In: DE Alexander and RW Fairbridge (eds) *Encyclopedia of Environmental Science*. Kluwer Academic Publishers, Hingham, MA.

7   Minami H and Tanaka K (1995) Social and environmental psychology: transaction between physical space and group dynamic processes. *Environ Behav.* **27**: 43–55.

8   Levine JM and Moreland RL (1998) Small groups. In: *The Handbook of Social Psychology*. McGraw-Hill, Boston, MA.

9   Brown BB and Perkins DD (1992) Disruptions in place attachments. In: E Altman and SM Low (eds) *Place Attachment*. Plenum, New York.

10   Maslow A (1968) *Towards a Psychology of Being*. Van Nostrand, New York.

11   Hall E (1966) *The Silent Language*. Doubleday, New York.

12   Alexander C, Ishikawa S and Silverstein MA (1977) *A Pattern Language*. Oxford University Press, New York.

13   Knowles MS (1980) *The Modern Practice of Adult Education: From Pedagogy to Andragogy*. Follet, Chicago.

14   Kindred M and Kindred M (1998) *Once Upon a Group...* 4M Publications, Southwell.

15   Brown G and Atkins M (1993) *Effective Teaching in Higher Education.* Routledge, London.

16   Bentley T (1993) *Facilitation: Providing Opportunities for Learning.* McGraw-Hill, London.

17   Justice T and Jamieson DW (1999) *The Facilitator's Fieldbook.* American Management Association Communications, AMA Publications, New York.

18   van Ments M (1989) *The Effective Use of Role Play.* Kogan Page, London.

19   Bourner T, Martin V and Race P (1993) *Workshops that Work: 100 Ideas to Make Your Training More Effective.* McGraw Hill Book Company, London.

4

Facilitation

> *Ralph lifted the conch. 'Seems to me we ought to have a chief to decide things.'*
> *'I ought to be chief', said Jack with simple arrogance.*
> *The dark boy, Roger, stirred at last and spoke up. 'Let's have a vote.'*
> William Golding, *Lord of the Flies*

What is facilitation?

Facilitating a group is not the same as leading it, nor is it a halfway house between acting as a group leader and participating as an ordinary member!

Box 4.1: Definition of facilitation

Facilitation is the work involved in ensuring that the right structures and processes exist for helping the group to meet its agreed objectives, and in helping the group members to identify and overcome problems in communicating with one another and in managing emotion.

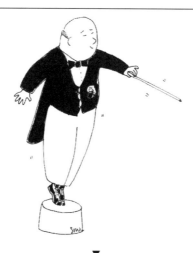

▼
What makes a good facilitator?

A facilitator has three overlapping tasks:

- to observe the group dynamics
- to manage the group process
- to obtain the best possible outcomes from the sum of the parts.

Although a facilitator is often thought of as someone 'external' who 'helps' a group, it is by no means impossible for groups to provide facilitation from within. However, most people do not possess the skills needed to facilitate groups, usually because they have never benefited from a neutral analysis of group dynamics. Furthermore, if the group is inexperienced, it may not have the level of maturity needed to allow one of its own members to take on the facilitator role, even if a suitable individual can be identified from within the group. In other words, facilitation can be performed by internal members *provided that*:

- the chosen member has the relevant skills and
- other members understand and respect the role difference.

Both participants (ordinary group members) and leaders must actively engage with the content of the group's task. They must contribute views, express opinions, make suggestions and shape the proposed group product. Facilitators should be as neutral as possible about the content issues, which is why internal facilitation can be awkward, particularly if an individual in a leadership position tries to 'facilitate' a group. Leaders who attempt to convey neutrality will always be distrusted. Conversely, facilitators who take positions on content issues within groups will lose their authority to manage the group process.

Although the benefits of groups and teams are well recognised, there are also common and significant problems that can severely limit their productivity. As we shall demonstrate in Chapter 10 (*see* p. 161), teams and groups can occasionally become dysfunctional and completely ineffective. However, it is more common to be involved in groups that have the predictable problems of interpersonal relationships. Even when it is not overtly dysfunctional, a group's ability to concentrate on the real issues can drift. Role confusion, misunderstandings, power rivalries, difficulties in achieving consensus, and lack of commitment to agreed actions are almost universal features of working in groups. Facilitation focuses on resolving these problems and ensures that the process enables problems to surface where necessary. Facilitation should also allow the correct resources and information to be available to ensure that the group's decision making is of the highest possible quality.

A facilitator must therefore take a very broad view of the task that faces the group, and must consider (and, if appropriate, delegate) the following three steps,[1] which are considered in more detail in Table 4.1.

Table 4.1:   Stages of facilitation

Stage 1 (preparatory work)	Stage 2 (group work)	Stage 3 (follow-up)
Agreeing the 'contract': look for details such as 'what, when and for how long' and, if relevant, 'financial considerations'	*Forming the group*: (for details, *see* p. 98). Think about the stages involved and plan exercises such as introductions, group charter or ground rules in order to establish group norms	*Evaluation*: this can be as simple as collecting 'happiness' indices or as complex as undertaking in-depth interviews with group members
Collecting data: make sure that you understand the culture and the context of the group you are to facilitate, and the broad nature of the task or objectives as perceived by the organisation	*Analysing the task*: make sure that you compare perceptions, and obtain and analyse information which is relevant to the task	*Consultation*: consider making an informal report to the organisation, agree the next steps and devise a schedule for reporting the results of the group work and any further actions that are required
Clarifying details: seek details about the group membership, leadership elements, external stakeholders, expected meeting structures and resources available for your use (information, time and/ or finance)	*Managing group dynamics*: conflict will always occur at some level, so be on the look-out to intervene when necessary to enhance performance, negotiate decision-making processes and increase group autonomy	*Reporting*: document the results of the group work in terms of process, outcomes and internal member participation (*see* Chapter 9)
Logistics: find out how to get information disseminated to group members, book rooms and equipment, arrange refreshments, and so on	*Closure*: even if a task has not been fully accomplished, it is important to reflect and evaluate the process. This will help to ensure clear action points for future meetings	*Actions*: Are there any actions that you need to take, either to address issues that were raised in the group or to secure further work within the organisation?

1   Preparatory work, which consists of:
   - defining who should be included in the group
   - identifying and consulting external stakeholders
   - considering whether the group's context and culture support the task and potential solutions
   - administration (e.g. sending out papers, booking rooms).
2   Group work, which consists of:
   - forming the group and setting ground rules
   - setting a climate of open, honest communication
   - helping the group to analyse the task
   - observing group dynamic and task achievement
   - maintaining participation and managing conflict

- achieving high-quality decision making, consensus and commitment to action.
3 Follow-up, which consists of:
  - evaluating the content and process of what went on
  - delivering the product.

Facilitation styles and dimensions

Facilitation styles are, in basic terms, situated somewhere along a spectrum ranging from highly directive to highly non-directive. Inexperienced facilitators tend to take refuge in one or other of these extremes. The non-directive facilitator's role is merely to 'be there', almost to the point of being a mute observer (or so it can seem). Although some groups can cope with this facilitation style and become autonomous relatively quickly, it can produce strong feelings of frustration and eventual protest among group members. On the other hand, the facilitator who has planned everything down to the last detail runs the risk of stifling all contributions. Introduce too much structure and the group will become dependent on scheduled exercises and discussions and fail to gain the autonomy required to maintain its stability and effectiveness.

John Heron's work,[2] building as it does on Carl Rogers' seminal book *Freedom to Learn*[3] and Malcolm Knowles' ideas on self-directed learning,[4] goes beyond a simple dichotomy into 'non-directive' and 'directive'. Heron described what he called three operational 'modes' of facilitation:

- *hierarchical mode* (consult the group, then *you* decide)
- *co-operative mode* (consult the group and then decide *with* them)
- *autonomous mode* (support the group – *they* decide).

In hierarchical mode, the facilitator is in control of the group and makes all of the major decisions. He or she determines the sequence of events, decides the objectives, interprets the process, and challenges or ignores resistance. This mode is often used when groups are meeting for the first time or are judged to be inexperienced at dealing with an interactive situation. Control provides security and can be reassuring when high levels of anxiety are expressed or perceived.

In co-operative mode, decision making is explicitly shared. The facilitator makes offers to the group about different components of the group process – structure, timing, interpretation of meaning and commentary on the feelings within the group – and guides and encourages members to negotiate decisions about the way in which they want to develop the interaction.

The autonomous mode is the most difficult form of facilitation to achieve successfully, and requires fine judgements about the capability of the group and its members. In this mode the facilitator respects the autonomy of the group – things are not done for them, or with them, but the freedom is provided for the group to make its own decisions without any external influence. A high level of understanding is required of the group process, especially when working with groups that are inexperienced in negotiating solutions openly, without hidden resistances. The goal is a self-directed, self-managing group that can maintain both an efficient task and a sustaining process.

Groups (and facilitators as they gain experience) usually move from hierarchical to autonomous modes of working, and the transitions have to be carefully managed. Facilitators who spend too long in a hierarchical mode or who never move from the co-operative to autonomous mode will foster feelings of both frustration and dependence.

Heron also suggested a further elaboration on the process of facilitation. He described six 'dimensions' or ways in which certain activities within groups could be categorised.

1   *The planning dimension.* How will the group's aims and objectives be achieved? What has to be done, how, and in what order, to achieve these goals? Planning can have a major influence on the group process, and should not be considered a purely administrative task.

2   *The meaning dimension.* How does the group 'understand' what is going on, i.e. how do they give meaning to the process in which they are participants? This normally requires a conscious distancing from both the content and task issues in order to reflect on the individual and group experiences.

3   *The confronting dimension.* Either as a collective or as individuals within groups, many important issues are often ignored or avoided. There are often complex reasons why these issues do not surface. This dimension considers the question of how, and to what end, the group becomes aware of the issues that it needs to face.

4   *The feeling dimension.* Strong feelings can be generated within groups, either of cohesion, camaraderie, loyalty and friendship, or conversely of irritation, anger and mistrust. Although groups will vary tremendously in the extent to which they focus consciously on feelings (e.g. psychodynamic support meeting vs. agenda-driven committee), they are ubiquitously present.

5   *The structuring dimension.* What form is given to experiences within the group (e.g. general discussion, role play, learning set techniques)?

6   *The valuing dimension.* Successful group work depends on open communication between individuals who respect each other's views and are prepared to enter a dialogue about the ways and means of making decisions and achieving goals. This form of interaction is almost impossible in a climate where people do not 'value' one another. This aspect of group work is, as Heron put it, about the creation of 'a supportive climate

in which members can be genuine, disclosing their reality as it is, keeping in touch with their true needs and interests'.

Effective facilitators are those who are able to move flexibly between different modes (hierarchical, co-operative, autonomous; *see* p. 52) and dimensions (planning, meaning, confronting, feeling, structuring, valuing; *see* p. 53) in the light of the changing group situations. The two grids shown in Table 4.2 illustrate how modes and dimensions can combine in different ways during a development process. This grid can be a useful tool for broadening the facilitative dimension, evaluating facilitation skills and monitoring development.

Table 4.2:   Analysing facilitation within a group process

At the start of a group process

	Planning	*Meaning*	*Confronting*	*Feeling*	*Structuring*	*Valuing*
Hierarchy	✓	✓	✓	✓	✓	✓
Co-operation						
Autonomy						

At the end of a group process

	Planning	*Meaning*	*Confronting*	*Feeling*	*Structuring*	*Valuing*
Hierarchy				✓		
Co-operation		✓	✓		✓	
Autonomy	✓					✓

Are good facilitators born or made?

The task of 'managing the process while remaining neutral about content' sounds deceptively simple. In practice, it is difficult and is often done badly. The skills required for effective facilitation have a sound theoretical basis which draws on adult learning theory (*see* p. 176),[4–7] group dynamics and decision making (*see* p. 238)[8] and process consultation (*see* p. 136).[9] The ability to apply these theoretical principles to the very practical task of running the group requires a particular set of personal qualities, including the following:

*   integrity, charisma and other aspects of personality that engender respect and trust from group members
*   insight and the ability to think quickly
*   flexibility generally, but assertiveness when the need arises

- optimism and realism in approximately equal doses (i.e. a positive but authentic attitude to any group's ability to achieve results)
- courage and honesty when difficult problems need to be surfaced and analysed.

Do not become too demoralised if you do not possess the 'full house' of these allegedly innate qualities of a good facilitator. Very few people do have them all! There is no doubt that many of the skills required for effective facilitation can be improved with experience and training,[1,2] including the ability to:

- manage time
- select appropriate venues and arrange the furniture to maximise effective communication within the group
- use a flipchart (*see* p. 46)
- design, explain and conduct structured exercises
- interpret behaviours, including non-verbal language ('body language')
- manage and confront interpersonal difficulties without inflaming the situation
- listen accurately and on behalf of others by asking for clarification
- help others to understand complex concepts
- modulate contributions to a group process by using the full range of communication skills, including physical movement around the group and the deployment of verbal and non-verbal cues.

Some individuals are much more skilled than others at remaining detached from the content of the group's work and concentrating on the process. This is not to say that the ability to relinquish control of content cannot be learned, but it does appear to be the most difficult aspect of this kind of work.[2] Facilitation helps to get things done, but people who 'want things done' often want it done *their* way, and hence naturally adopt the role of leader or vocal group member. If you know that you tend to do this, you would be doing your group a favour if you held back from volunteering to facilitate!

Facilitation techniques

The techniques and interventions of successful facilitation have been well described, and are summarised in Table 4.3.[1,10,11] A facilitator needs to have an acute sense of personal awareness and sensitivity to the surrounding processes. Heron called these qualities 'being *here* now' and 'being *there* now', endowing them with almost mystical importance. By being unencumbered by external thoughts or distracting anxieties, a facilitator is able to give complete and energising attention to the group. This quality of attentiveness is difficult to describe, but its presence (or absence) is immediately evident from their gaze, posture, movement, pace, intonation and speech content.[12] Expert facilitators are usually uniquely attentive yet also relaxed.

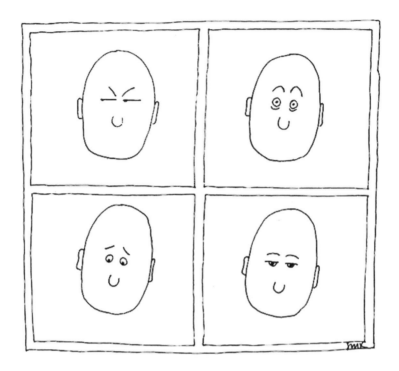

▼

The subtle use of eye contact.

Table 4.3:   Facilitation skills

Attentiveness	Concentrated awareness of self and surrounding activities, a state of relaxed alertness
Eye contact	Using scanning techniques to be aware of who wishes to contribute and using gaze to control the intensity and duration of participation
Movement and gesture	Making subtle use of the classic 'traffic officer' gesture to help to end a contribution and allow others to enter. Using movement (either spatial or by gesture) towards or away from group member to create interaction
Echoing	Repeating phrases as an indirect way of questioning. This technique (which is also used in contexts such as psychotherapy and non-directive counselling) conveys interest and attention, and moreover can beckon further thought, without influencing a particular train of thought. Echoing works best when done without an interrogative tone, and when phrases are reflected as accurately as possible. This technique can of course be used selectively, to emphasise and explore specific areas

Table 4.3:   Continued

Questions – open and closed	Closed questions elicit short and specific answers, and there is usually only one right answer. Condensing queries and searching for correct answers leads to closed questioning and will restrain participation. Open questions allow more scope for disclosure; informants will choose to answer in differing ways which will reflect their own thought processes. The distinction is not absolute, and people will vary in the way that they interpret questions. Forming open questions is not easy if anxiety or stress causes a facilitator to become concerned about 'helping' a group to achieve a predetermined objective
Leading or following	A facilitator who is employing the hierarchical mode (*see* p. 52) will use 'leading' questions in order to direct the group process. Questions which gently 'follow' the issues raised, and elicit more depth or other perspectives, will usually reduce the pace of events and allow the group to develop a sense of self-determination. The balance between and the timing of these types of probes will largely determine the facilitation style
Exploring the depths	Facilitators need to decide when (and when not) to explore the hidden aspects of interactions. For example, when a member of the group says 'that's all I can say about this', it is unlikely to be a true statement. If a decision is made to explore this contribution in greater depth, it is generally better to make statements rather than to make judgements. Using phrases such as 'You seem to be reluctant to say more about this...' should be combined with gestures and tone that signal empathy. Picking up on non-verbal cues can be a powerful intervention. Silences should only be interrupted by using the open question, 'What are you thinking?'. Facilitators need to use these techniques judiciously, and should beware of hunting for issues or conflicts that suit their own ends
Checking and formulating meaning	This technique should be used sparingly, as it can undermine participation levels, but it can help at those times when a contribution is poorly formulated. Interjecting a phrase such as 'I'm not sure if I've understood, you're saying that...' and then immediately providing a summarised version allows the individual concerned to confirm or reject the interpretation. This can also be done at a more global level, summarising vocal interactions ('It seems that the two of you disagree about...') and checking your interpretation with the group as a whole
Emphasis and structure	The facilitator can choose to emphasise selected issues by summarising or repeating (e.g. paraphrasing) important contributions. Providing structure (e.g. drawing together related elements, pointing to inconsistencies and organising the group process into identifiable sections) helps a group to reflect on its progress and make decisions about the next steps
Timekeeping	Meticulous adherence to starting and finishing times is essentially a form of modelling. By keeping to agreed times, the facilitator is publicly fulfilling their part of the contract and performing one of the most visible elements of the facilitation process. Agree on major time milestones at the start of the session (e.g. we break for coffee here, we allow half an hour at the end to discuss achievements and five minutes to agree on our work for the next session)

Table 4.3: Continued from previous page

Time out	The term 'time out' is borrowed from baseball procedures to refer to calling a halt to events. In a small group setting it is used to raise the group's awareness of process when they are excessively focused on content. The facilitator (or indeed any member of the group) may call a 'time out' by using directive body language (raising the hands in the shape of a 'T') to block the flow of conversation, thereby raising awareness of the 'metasituation', i.e. getting the members to focus on 'what's going on [in our interactions and assumptions] here'. At times the technique can seem contrived and intrusive, and if used too often it can become an irritant. An example of the use of this technique is given in Chapter 9 (*see* p. 150).

Dealing with 'difficult' group members

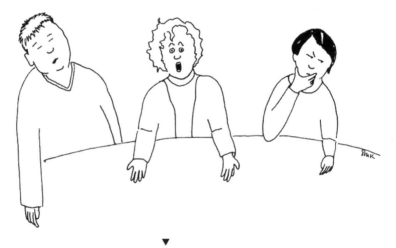

▼
Difficult group members.

We need to be extremely careful when we label behaviours as destructive or difficult. It is often the case that those who are disturbing the group dynamic are correct to do so. Apathy, unchallenged assumptions and uncritical acceptance of group norms and decisions often lie at the heart of poor group performance (*see* p. 161). However, it is clear that in many groups varying levels of motivations and interest can be found and challenging behaviours may be frequent. Several examples are listed below.

1   Some individuals may talk too much, including:
   • the dominator (*see* Box 4.2)
   • the enthusiast (*see* Box 4.3)
   • the conferrer (*see* Box 4.4).

2   Some may talk inappropriately, including:
    •   the digressor (*see* Box 4.5)
    •   the debater (*see* Box 4.6)
    •   the know-all (*see* Box 4.7)
    •   the joker (*see* Box 4.8).
3   Some may hardly talk at all, including:
    •   the timid (or reticent) member (*see* Box 4.9)
    •   the passive aggressor (*see* Box 4.10).
4   Some may show other forms of potentially destructive behaviour:
    •   the whinger (*see* Box 4.11)
    •   the rank-puller (*see* Box 4.12)
    •   the politician (*see* Box 4.13)
    •   the neurotic (*see* Box 4.14).

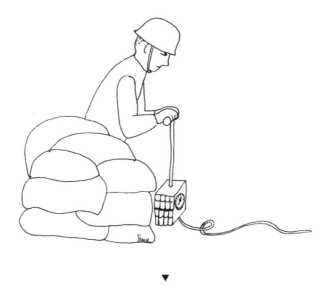

▼

We need to be careful when we label behaviours as destructive.

It is important to distinguish between personality (by definition, the aspects of personhood that are difficult or impossible to change) and behaviours that are limited to a particular situation or context (which will be more amenable to change). You are probably very aware of what type of personality you have (e.g. whether you are extrovert or introvert, sensitive or thick-skinned, and so on). Personality is composed of a number of component traits which, in certain combinations, produce what the group may perceive as a 'type' (*see* Table 4.4).

Table 4.4: Examples of trait attributes and resulting perceptions of those attributes in a social context

	Extrovert			Introvert		
	'The politician'	'The joker'	'The bully'	'The brain'	'The guru'	'The neurotic'
Ambitious	●	○				
Self-assured	●	○				
Diplomatic	●	○				
Boisterous	●	○				
Charismatic	○	●				
Extroverted	○	●				
Entertaining	○	●				
Exuberant		●				
Lively		●				
Spirited		●				
Silly		●				
Argumentative			●			
Manipulative			●			
Domineering			●			
Bullying			●			
Harassing			●			
Harsh			●			
Tough			●			
Glib			●			
Brainy				●	○	
Studious				●	○	
Intelligent				●	○	
Contemplative				○	●	
Meditative				○	●	
Introspective				○	●	
Inhibited						●
Shy						●
Withdrawn						●
Introverted						●
Melancholy						●
Self-conscious						●

●, main defining traits; ○, associated traits.

Sources: Handy C (1993) Perceiving people. In: *Understanding Organisations* (4e). Penguin, Harmondsworth.

Anderson SM and Klatsky RL (1987) Traits and social stereotypes: levels of categorisation in social perception. *J Person Soc Psychol.* **53**: 235–46.

Dealing with a particular extreme personality can be challenging, but note that the 'types' in Table 4.4 refer to what the group perceives (i.e. they are stereotypes) rather than what the individual necessarily represents. A person whose behaviour is interpreted by the group as characteristic of 'the bully' is likely to be more of a problem than someone whose behaviour is perceived as representing 'the guru'. Boxes 4.2 to 4.14 show some additional 'types' whose behaviour can potentially derail the group process.

Box 4.2:   The dominator

This person talks whenever there is a chance, usually at great length if not in depth, and you can spot the resignation and the raised eyebrows among other group members. It can be difficult to curb this behaviour during group work.
   To manage this behaviour:

- make a well-timed sensitive private request for the individual to allow others to contribute
- recognise and privately praise their efforts at self-awareness
- direct questions to other members by eye contact or name
- acknowledge the contribution quickly and ask for other views
- ask the individual to take on a task which requires attention to detail, such as writing detailed records to provide feedback to a plenary session.

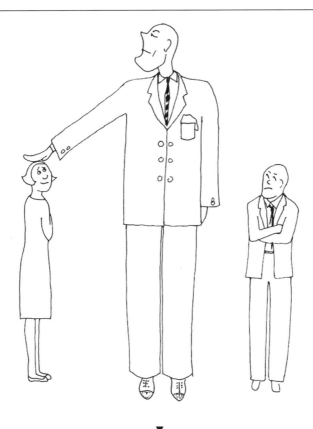

▼

The dominator.

Box 4.3: The enthusiast

This individual is knowledgeable, keen and extrovert. They often anticipate questions and are ahead of the group. Although this type of behaviour can be an asset when things are slow to get off the ground, it can also inhibit others because they take more time to become engaged. The enthusiast, like the dominator, needs to become aware of others.

To manage this behaviour:

- avoid commenting on the enthusiast's reply, but look at others expectantly
- announce that you are interested in a range of responses
- ask questions of others by means of nods or eye contact.

Box 4.4: The conferrer

This individual turns to colleagues and confers, to share either a comment, a quip or a criticism. The group is never included and indeed feels excluded. There is often a conspiracy afoot and a pair or triad will arrange to sit together. Sometimes other members are pulled into these private conversations and find it difficult to resist the invitation to share confidences. At the most basic level, this type of behaviour is disrespectful of the group process.

To manage this behaviour:

- use pauses and body language to listen in to the 'conference'
- check whether the private conversation can contribute to the wider discussion
- change the group's seating positions regularly
- confront the conferrer directly, pointing out the disrespectful nature of the interruption.

The use of humour may help to defuse this type of situation.

Box 4.5: The disgressor

Although digressions can be extremely useful and illuminating, the person who always describes the perfect tangent can frustrate the discussion, waste time and turn a constructive event into a fruitless argument.

To manage this behaviour:

- use time pressure (e.g. 'that's an interesting point, but we're a bit pushed for time at the moment...')
- point out the digression and make an explicit decision, with the involvement of the group if necessary, as to whether to follow this tangent or to pull the group back to the main point.

This latter technique has the effect of letting the group know that you are not willing to let other agendas sabotage the main issues. However, it can be seen as a controlling mechanism and therefore needs to be used with discretion.

Box 4.6: The debater

There are occasions when a vigorous informed debate can be exciting and rewarding, and being part of such a discussion is a privilege. However, there are people who like to debate irrelevant details, dwell on semantics and set up battles in order to either impress or digress.

To manage this behaviour:

• gently assert that 'in order to move on, let's agree to disagree on this issue'
• interject by agreeing that they are making a valid point, but that you would like to hear from others whether this is an important issue
• use humour to suggest that this is such an important point that it needs at least two hours, which you will happily spend on it after the group work has been completed.

Box 4.7: The know-all

This individual often uses jargon, name-drops and assumes that others have the same knowledge base. Beneath the veneer, they may have an immature or insecure personality.

To manage this behaviour:

• establish a rule that it is important to clarify the use of new terms or ideas, and illustrate this principle by interjecting immediately
• encourage an ethos where the responsibility to learn is a shared objective, by providing explanations and pointers to new sources of information
• question assumptions and expertise, and assert the view that claiming 'knowledge' brings with it a responsibility to share it with others.

Box 4.8: The joker

Humour can often motivate a group, but some individuals use the clown role as a deliberate or subconscious wrecking tactic. Their contributions, instead of oiling the wheels of intergroup communication, are invariably frivolous, stupid, sexist or even racist, and may undermine hours of concerted work.

To manage this behaviour:

• reward the individual's non-frivolous contributions
• gently reject the quip and ask for views on the issue in hand
• confront the individual outside the group.

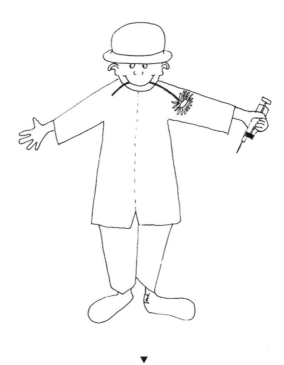

▼

The joker with an injection of light relief.

Box 4.9:   The timid (or reticent) member

The reticent member may be very comfortable with that role, so beware of making assumptions that he or she needs to be 'brought in'. Truly 'timid' individuals worry about the 'how' or the 'what' (or both) of their contributions. Because they often lack self-confidence, they are usually extremely attentive, and will be able to take on summarisation tasks or provide reflections on process with great accuracy. Asking shy members to take on these roles at an early stage enables a gradual entry into the group activity. There are also techniques that can be used which help to ensure participation.

   To manage this behaviour:

- use the shy member productively (e.g. in note-taking or timekeeping – introverts tend to relish such non-threatening ways of participating in the group)
- when tasks or questions are set, ask each member to write a short list of ideas or thoughts. The facilitator can then use a range of methods to harvest the suggestions and therefore ensure that the contributions of the timid members are given attention
- use pairs or buzz groups (*see* p. 79) to assist the integration of the shy member, particularly if the group activities are dynamic and involve making new relationships in less exposed situations.

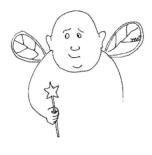

▼
The timid or reticent member.

Box 4.10: The passive aggressor

This individual is one of the most destructive types of all to have within a group, because of their inhibitory effect on others. By sitting still and declining to nod, smile or acknowledge any group activity, the presence of this quiet member will soon pervade the general mood of the group. One of the most important functions of the first three steps of forming a group process (introduction, ground rules and ice-breaking; *see* Chapter 6, p. 97) is to make it explicit that this type of behaviour does not become the norm for the group process.

If the individual persists in adopting a negative passive attitude, it is a matter of facilitator style and experience whether to:

- ignore the member or
- confront them, either within or outside the group dynamic.

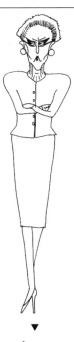

▼
The passive aggressor.

Box 4.11: The whinger

This individual is adept at finding fault and is not afraid to complain or attribute blame. Relentless whinging can be very difficult to handle, especially when there is support for the criticism in the group. It is inevitable that there will be faults in any course or workshop. Practical problems, unforeseen gaps in content and mishaps in process will occur even in the best circumstances. It is often counter-productive to defend a criticism within the group process unless this can become part of your evaluation process. Acknowledging criticism, asking for specific descriptions and asking for constructive suggestions for achieving improvement on the next occasion is an honest and useful method of dealing with a well-founded criticism. However, there are critics who like to grouse about less important problems.

To manage this behaviour:

- ask the group to 'comment on X's point'
- ask the group for permission to move on
- confront the individual outside the group.

Box 4.12: The rank-puller

This individual generally holds high status outside the group and attempts to use this to challenge the internal leadership. The situation becomes even more complex if the rank-puller has subordinates who are participating in the group itself. The key to handling this type of behaviour is a combination of anticipation and honesty.

To manage this behaviour:

- the facilitator may want to discuss the effect of high status on the group process with the individual concerned before the work starts, and explain the potential pitfalls for the individual, the group and the facilitator
- the same can be done within the group process itself, but this is a much more risky approach; one way of tackling it is to consider the effect of 'status' on the weight given to contributions in the ground-rule setting exercise (*see* Chapter 6)
- the use of humour to point up the high rank in order to neutralise its effect.

Box 4.13: The politician

This individual works hard during the early phases of the group to ingratiate him- or herself gently with as many people as possible, usually by means of compliments and *bonhomie*, although such behaviour may at times appear to be transparent and superficial. The politician assesses interests within the group and calculates the position that will maximise their own advantage, usually for

continued opposite

personal but sometimes for organisational gain. The politician is metaphoric-
ally the last to vote, and waits until the direction has been clearly decided before
contributing a view. Their aim is to survive, to be on the winning team, and if
necessary to manipulate.

To manage this behaviour:

- accept that some people are politicians and learn the skills!
- if manipulation of subgroups is obvious and disruptive, use the techniques
  of agenda setting and nominal groups to clear the air
- use the technique of 'reverse argument position' and ask individuals
  (including the politician) to state the alternative positions.

Box 4.14:   The neurotic

This individual is a worrier, and is forever raising the spectre of 'what might
happen if', or generally raising the anxiety of the group by sharing anxieties
about personal or group performance. The issues are not usually mission-
critical, but more often to do with small details or tangents, such as false
deadlines or concerns about the 'crockery'.

To manage this behaviour:

- recognise the concerns but ask for permission to 'park' them for the
  moment, so that they can be addressed at an agreed time – preferably a few
  minutes before an agreed break for coffee
- agree to spend time tackling concerns and anxieties at a fixed point in the
  group session, but only after the major decisions have been agreed and good
  processes are in place
- use humour, but be careful not to humiliate the individual concerned.
  Woody Allen-like characters engender a lot of sympathy, and you could get
  caught up in a group backlash.

The behaviours shown in Boxes 4.2 to 4.14 are in many respects 'normal',
but they can impede both the development of the group process and
the potential learning that can take place. It is important to avoid superficial stereotyping or jumping to conclusions. For example, there are many
different types of quiet contributor, each of which poses a very different
challenge. Some choose not to contribute, while others wish that they had
the courage to do so, and often do not realise the potential value of their
contribution.

There are disadvantages to the facilitator taking on the task of confronting
destructive behaviours. Groups may feel threatened by the intervention, or
they may become dependent on external leadership. Nevertheless, there are

occasions when a facilitator needs to take control merely in order to preserve a constructive environment. This is particularly true for groups that only have a brief lifespan, and which are therefore unable to work through their 'storming' phase, where issues of control and inclusion could be addressed organically. Boxes 4.2 to 4.14 suggest specific tactics for dealing with each example of difficult behaviour, but the reader should note that the suggested techniques must be used sparingly and with subtlety.

With all difficult behaviours it can be very instructive to take time to analyse the following questions.

- What effect is the difficult group member having on you, and how are you responding?
- How is the difficult group member affecting others in the group?
- Does the individual get a pay-off for their difficult behaviour?
- Is there an explanation for their behaviour?

Group members may have supplied clues to the underlying reason for their difficult behaviour during introductions and successive contributions. Using coffee breaks to explore the views of the individual concerned about the group's activities and how they relate to personal aims may provide additional insights. The following questions serve as examples.

- Is the individual bent on destroying the group? This is unusual.
- Is the individual in the group under duress (e.g. on an imposed and unwanted training course)?
- Do they usually have an elevated status outside the group?
- Has a previous negative experience coloured their approach to working in groups?
- Do they lack basic interpersonal skills? What can you do about that?
- What other events in their lives may be acting as a distraction or source of irritation?

Table 4.5 outlines the methods that can help to change or at least subdue difficult behaviour. However, it is important to beware of trying to achieve too much within the group dynamic, and to look for opportunities to try to resolve this type of disruptive behaviour on a one-to-one basis.

Giving and receiving feedback

It is important to follow the rules of feedback (the guidelines given below are partly based on the 'Pendleton rules')[13] so that the process is both effective and respected. Note that although facilitators are generally keen to avoid an excessive focus on 'negative' points, there are times when it is important not to shy away from providing information about poor performance or aspects

Table 4.5:   General strategies for addressing difficult behaviour

Let the group challenge the behaviour	If an individual is preventing the group from working, it is unlikely that the facilitator is the only one who is feeling frustrated. Use the confronting dimension to enable group members to challenge individuals who are being difficult. This opportunity for challenge can be created in a variety of ways. The use of 'time out/time in' breaks (*see* p. 150) to reflect on 'process' is a powerful, if occasionally intrusive, technique
Use eye contact and body language	If sustained eye contact is not sufficient to allow a pause of contribution, body language signals such as raising a hand gently usually provide an adequate signal, especially for the enthusiastic but benign over-contributor
Split the group	This is useful in situations where pairs or cliques have formed that are running separate dialogues. By the time that the group is brought back together, the original dynamic will usually have changed, especially if seating is altered
Share the burden and test for consensus	If one member of the group attacks your strategy, beware of spending time as a leader-facilitator defending in detail why you have chosen to include such-and-such an exercise, unless of course you accept the critique and adapt your plans accordingly. Share the attack with the group and check for consensus. A good facilitator can gauge the group support and abandon fixed plans if necessary. Justifying your actions leaves you vulnerable to counter-arguments, whereas if you explain why you chose to adopt a particular strategy, this puts you in a much more neutral and honest position. It is easier to change your plans if you avoid defending a position

which could be improved. We have found the following ten 'rules' particularly useful when running feedback sessions.

Make time for feedback

Make sure that adequate and protected space is left for feedback, and that both the designated individual and the group as a whole are aware that this is both planned and essential – not an afterthought which is only included when a 'poor' performance needs urgent attention.

Use a set order with priority given to the individual

Convention holds that the order for feedback in a small group is as follows:

- the individual, who should first suggest the things that went well and then consider the things they would like to do differently next time

- the group members
- the facilitator.

Avoid scoring points

Remember that feedback says a lot about you as well as about the person to whom it is directed. Ask yourself 'Why am I giving this feedback?'. Is it to demonstrate something about yourself? Or is it to help the person concerned improve their own performance? If you want to show how much you know, or contribute generally to the topic under discussion, the feedback session is not the place to do this.

Be constructive

It should be obvious that the vital part of the feedback process is to work on ways of improving future performances, by making specific suggestions and, if necessary, allowing repeated rehearsals. It is not enough to describe the faults or weaknesses. The classic question used is 'If you were to do it again, what would you change or improve, and how?' It is within this reframing process that reflection and active learning takes place. When the group or individual has completed these basic feedback tasks, there is usually surprisingly little for others to add.

Make observations, not assumptions

Avoid declaring your opinions or assigning motives (e.g. 'You were trying to intimidate her'). Instead, try to describe specific behaviours and give examples (e.g. 'You stood up and spoke loudly'). If relevant, you could draw out motives by asking the individual for his or her views on your observations.

Give reactions, not judgements

It is particularly important not to speak on behalf of others when you are providing feedback. Do not use expressions that contain the phrase 'we felt...', but speak about your own feelings without making judgements. For instance, say 'When you raised your voice at that point, I felt anxious', rather than

'We all thought that you had become angry and were in danger of losing control'.

Give specific examples, not general impressions

This is important for both positive and negative behaviours. It is easy to describe an encounter as 'friendly but professional', but far more rewarding to say 'Your handshake was firm and of the correct duration, and you managed to direct me to the most appropriate seat without making me feel awkward'. It will be much easier for someone to emulate the 'friendly and professional' role if they understand the components.

Concentrate on what is possible and most important

Confine your comments to things that can be changed. There is no point in saying 'You've got a very difficult accent to understand', but you could say 'I think your presentation would be improved if you spoke more slowly and repeated your key points'. For example, a novice who is struggling to present a summary of a research paper should not be given feedback about their inability to process the finer points of the statistical analysis. A far better use of the feedback session would be to help them to realise that the research method chosen was not the most ideal one for the question posed.

Use questions, not suggestions

Experienced facilitators will be adept at the use of questions that help individuals to conceptualise solutions for themselves. Questions such as 'What other ways could there be of reacting in that situation? Let's think them through...' can be used. This approach is far more effective than the use of phrases such as 'You should have done this...'.

Don't be overwhelming

Feedback is best provided within an established tutor–student or facilitator–group relationship, and this is normally done in steps that are small and frequent. As a rule, one or two 'negative' areas are the maximum that can be successfully handled within a feedback session, especially during the early stages. So stop before the shutters go up.

References

1   Justice T and Jamieson DW (1999) *The Facilitator's Fieldbook*. American Management Association Communications, AMA Publications, New York.

2   Heron J (1989) *The Facilitator's Handbook*. Kogan Page, London.

3   Rogers C (1983) *Freedom to Learn for the Eighties*. Charles E Merrill, Columbus, OH.

4   Knowles MS (1980) *The Modern Practice of Adult Education: From Pedagogy to Andragogy*. Follet, Chicago.

5   Rogers A (1986) *Teaching Adults*. Open University Press, Milton Keynes.

6   Gagne RM (1985) *The Conditions of Learning and Theory of Instruction* (4e). Holt-Sanders, New York.

7   Brookfield SD (1986) *Understanding and Facilitating Adult Learning*. Open University Press, Buckingham.

8   Levine JM and Moreland RL (1998) Small groups. In: *The Handbook of Social Psychology*. McGraw-Hill, Boston, MA.

9   Schein E (1988) *Process Consultation* (2e). Addison-Wesley, Reading, MA.

10   Jaques D (1984) *Learning in Groups*. Kogan Page, London.

11   Heron J (1989) *Six Category Intervention Analysis. Human Potential Research Project* (3e). University of Surrey, Guildford.

12   Argyle M (1994) *The Psychology of Interpersonal Behaviour* (5e). Penguin, Harmondsworth.

13   Pendleton D, Schofield T, Tate P and Havelock P (1984) *The Consultation: an Approach to Learning and Teaching*. Oxford University Press, Oxford.

5

Methods used in group work

Individual work and personality assessment

There are considerable advantages to beginning small group work by concentrating on the actual individuals involved. The principle of 'know thyself'

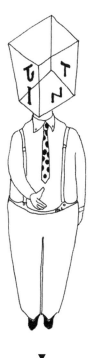

▼

'How d'you do, I'm an INTJ.'

is fundamental to understanding how an individual reacts both to others and to tasks that involve different levels of skills and participation. This process can of course take many forms, and can vary in complexity. For instance, Box 5.1 describes a method that can help individuals to focus on their personal journeys and the influences that have shaped their personalities. It can be undertaken at varying levels of depth, and is probably best reserved for groups that are going to remain stable and in close working relationships for a lengthy period of time.

Box 5.1:   Drawing a life-line

Drawing a life-line on a piece of plain paper (showing high and low points) and mapping out key events is a simple way for individuals to reflect on their personal development and probable future direction. The extent to which people share their diagrams can be tailored to the time and aims of the exercise. Be warned that this process can take much longer than you think (allow 20–30 minutes per person), and be ready to handle personal distress. It is vital to have agreed very 'safety' oriented ground rules before this exercise is performed.

Being sensitive to diversity

Even in the most homogeneous of groups there will be striking degrees of diversity – in views, style of dress, attitudes and personality. It is this very mix and contrast that provides groups with their energy and the potential for tremendous conflict, which sometimes occurs unexpectedly. Exposing elements of this diversity can be extremely threatening to individuals, as people fear that their worst features will be revealed, their insecurities, prejudices and gaps in knowledge and skills exposed, and occasionally even darker or more painful problems revealed. Individuals sometimes feel an impulse to share such feelings in a small group context, perhaps hoping for a shared understanding. This is not to deny that groups can provide support, but it is also a common experience that revelations of this type may be deeply regretted, cause embarrassment all round and significantly disrupt the group's confidence and atmosphere of safety, especially if the group is new and exploratory.

We therefore recognise that, although it may be important to consider analysing personality and personal characteristics in some depth, this needs to be done with a constant monitoring of personal boundaries, and by stressing the risks and benefits of self-disclosure.

There are many different ways in which personality can be analysed. Two main themes dominate the personality theory literature, namely the internal and external influences on individuals. Sigmund Freud and others in the psychoanalytical tradition, particularly Jung, developed the 'internal' thread – that is, the influences of the 'conscious, preconscious and unconscious mind'. Alfred Adler examined the concept of personality from perspectives such as birth order (ideas of worth) and feelings of 'superiority' (hence the idea that some people have 'inferiority complexes'). In the 1960s, Isabel Briggs Myers (see below) developed the Jungian concept that a typology of personalities exists. However, there are other perfectly valid ways of looking at personality. Cognitivists spawned the term 'learned helplessness', that view being that our cognitive structures (negative and positive) determine how we behave.

Skinner preferred to downplay the 'internal' influences and adopted the archetypal behaviourist approach by suggesting that it is bells, whistles and food that operate to condition our lives.[1] More recently, Bandura[2] and others (social-cognitive and social constructionist theorists) have stressed that it is much more likely that 'personalities' are a complex weave of all of these facets (*see* Box 5.2).

Box 5.2:   Bandura and the 'bobo dolls'

Bandura is famous for reporting the 'bobo doll' studies. He filmed a young female student beating up an inflatable doll (weighted so that it automatically reverted to the upright position) by shouting, kicking and using a hammer. The film was shown to groups of young children, who (predictably) liked it. They were then shown a playroom in which, included among other play items, were a 'bobo doll' and hammers. Many of the children immediately assaulted the doll and imitated the behaviours precisely, using similar words and actions.

Bandura observed that the children changed their behaviours without first being rewarded for approximations to that behaviour. In other words, this did not fit so well with standard behaviouristic learning theory. Bandura called this phenomenon 'observational learning' or 'modelling', and his theory is usually referred to as social learning theory.

Goleman has more recently proposed the idea that 'emotional intelligence' exists,[3] and that it is one of the key determinants of success in life! True or not, this very brief overview illustrates the complexity of this area, and although we shall focus attention in this chapter on two very well-known instruments, a web search will locate a myriad of other readily available personality tests.

A popular exercise in management training is to calculate the Belbin 'team role' types (*see* Chapter 16, p. 261).[4] Understanding that you are a group of leader types who are always having good ideas and writing proposals, but who lack individuals who can make notes, obtain resources and arrange meetings may help to explain why high expectations often seem to lead to a succession of disappointments. If groups are to work together for any sustained

Introversion	I	Reflective, internalised methods of interacting with others
Extroversion	E	Energy flows outwards, participates easily and acts quickly

Sensing	S	Understands details and facts, likes the practical, the 'here and now'
Intuition	N	Prefers thinking about patterns, concepts and the future

Thinking	T	Objective, analytical and impersonal
Feeling	F	Subjective, personal, and deals with emotions and values

Judgement	J	Decisive, sets limits and establishes closure
Perception	P	Curious, discursive and maintains open exploration

Figure 5.1:   The four dimensions in the Myers-Briggs Personality Type Inventory.

period of time, it may be worth considering using a personality inventory, such as the Myers-Briggs Type Indicator. This was devised by Isabel Briggs Myers and her mother, Katherine Briggs, and was originally based on Jung's theory of psychological types. There are four dimension pairs along which personality type preferences are assigned (*see* Figure 5.1). A total of 16 different combinations are therefore described, and are abbreviated by the assigned letters in the second column of Figure 5.1.

While working on this book, we each worked out our own Myers-Briggs type (there are now self-administered questionnaires available on the Internet if you are interested in finding your own type).[5] Glyn Elwyn and Sian Koppel are INTJs (introversion, intuition, thinking and judgement). Trisha Greenhalgh is ESTJ (extroversion, sensing, thinking and judgement) and Fraser Macfarlane is ISFJ (introversion, sensing, feeling and judgement). As many people at the INSEAD Business School programme in 1999 remarked about the inventory when they determined their personality type, it can be frighteningly accurate! However, it also has to be recognised that there are 'types' who hate being 'typed' (or 'traited'), so you should be ready to defend, or at least explain, your chosen analysis method.

Apart from providing a good basis for comparing notes and asking those who know you well how close the fit is, conducting this exercise will also reveal the Achilles' heel of your personality type, which Myers and Briggs term 'the grip'. For example, for an INTJ the grip consists of a severe narrowing of the ability to take a wide view, an obsessive focus on external data, over-indulgence in sensual pleasure and an adversarial attitude towards the outer world. When we find one of this book's authors arguing about the minutiae of the project (and raiding the refrigerator for cheese late at night), we can at least understand that this is an aspect of personality. If you decide to include a Myers-Briggs Type Inventory as part of your group experience, you will need to be in the hands of an experienced facilitator who has negotiated access to the full range of associated literature.[6,7]

Choosing methods

In this chapter and elsewhere (*see* Chapters 6, 7, 8 and 14) a wide range of methods, techniques and exercises is described. Choosing the correct method to use can often be as difficult as executing the work. Although first-hand experience will inevitably guide the way in which you construct your small group work sessions, the following guidelines are designed to help you to avoid the most obvious problems that can occur.

Forming a small group in the middle of a day's course is a very different task to being responsible for a course that lasts a whole week. Other groups meet for small amounts of time but may do so for many years (e.g. committees and project teams). Facilitators therefore have to think extremely carefully about the degree of explicitness, group honesty, the size of the task and the evolution of appropriate team roles.

Short lifespan groups

These groups are typically given an hour or less for meetings. They are one of the most difficult types of group to handle, and very often fail because the individuals involved are unclear about the task and how to fulfil it, do not have any rapport with one another, and are frequently frustrated by the apparent irrelevance of the exercise. It is therefore critically important not to inflame the (often hidden) frustration by introducing additional talks that have the potential to cause irritation. The use of time-consuming or simplistic ice-breakers should be avoided. If the group has an unclear task, make it your first duty as a facilitator to achieve clarity, even if this requires a fairly direct-ive approach. 'Introductions' and 'ground-rule setting' (*see* pp. 98 and 102) should not be omitted, but they need to be compressed into the minimum amount of time. Explaining and obtaining permission to use a fast way of covering these tasks can help to set the tone and increase the productivity of the group. The use of masking tape to generate name labels is both an ice-breaking activity (especially if it involves sharing a roll of tape and some pens) and also quickly achieves the goal of matching names to faces. If each person is asked to specify one ground rule within a 3-minute guillotine, after you have first written up three obvious and pertinent ones, this can get the process off to a good start. It rapidly sets the scene, indicates that you mean business and helps the participants understand that to achieve results, the whole group needs to react quickly and efficiently.

The week-long group

Courses that last for a week or more usually involve people who have been drawn together from many different parts of the country, and at least one session should be devoted entirely to getting to know each other's personal objectives and agreeing a rough outline of content and process for the week. These aims should be explicitly re-negotiated at regular intervals. It is often possible to achieve a great deal of honesty in groups that have a limited time-frame, and the Johari window (*see* p. 164) and other self-disclosure techniques can be used to obtain levels of personal feedback that are often very difficult to achieve in work environments or other more stable contexts. Facilitators should be brave enough to explore these methods and skilled enough to support the inevitable (and sometimes painful) personal journeys and insights that occur.

Recurring groups with a long timespan

It is often assumed that these groups do not need to examine their internal processes. Committees, boards and project teams are often aware that group dynamics are either contributing to or hindering their work, but are typically unable or unprepared to consider these areas in any real depth. However, it is clear that 'away-days' and 'team-development' workshops are being increasingly used to explore such interactions. Choosing methods for these events is a matter of matching the exercise to the aim. It should not be assumed that a mature group process has been established. All groups will have formed 'norms', as this stage occurs quickly and inevitably (*see* p. 119), but the degree to which 'storms' and role conflicts have been resolved will vary. Extensive introductions and ice-breaking techniques will be irrelevant for a well-established group, but insights into personality preferences will be both entertaining and relevant to people who have to establish and maintain long working relationships. Role clarification and listening exercises will reveal tension about how decisions are made, and games and simulations that explore the 'dark side' of group decision-making processes will be highly relevant (*see* p. 83). The model of situational leadership will be highly relevant (*see* p. 278), and the techniques of conflict resolution described in Chapter 8 should be used whenever a group becomes 'stuck'. Groups that have become complacent and tired, or which are unable to see that their structure is preventing new developments, should regularly try formal brainstorming and nominal group methods, both to regenerate the group and to give voice to those who may find it difficult to influence the power dynamic assumptions that have been generated over time.

Pairs and triads ('buzz groups')

Research into small group formation indicates that all groups are in effect combinations of pairs and triads. These comprise the basic unit of close interaction between people. Facilitators of small groups often make use of these units to increase levels of participation. They are commonly called 'buzz groups' – a reference to the noise and activity that can be witnessed in a room when a large group is divided in this way.

The task should be easily understood but not trivial, and it is best if the amount of physical movement required is minimal. It is normal to ask people to turn to their immediate neighbours. If the layout allows chairs to be moved, ask group members to rearrange their chairs so that individuals turn to face each other. The discussion should not take more than a few minutes, and it is best to pull the whole group together long before the 'buzz' dies down. Incidentally, this technique can also be used in larger groups, such as a group in a lecture hall, and will increase the ability of the audience both to concentrate and to become involved. Such an approach has also been cynically described as the facilitator's last resort, so beware of the repeated use of the command 'turn to your neighbour'.

Snowballing

Snowballing (and pyramiding) describe the technique of amalgamating buzz groups into progressively larger groups until the whole group comes together again in a plenary session. This method is particularly effective if buzz groups have structured tasks which they have to then agree or build on as the units increase in size. Performing the same task repetitively can lead to boredom or irritation, and careful attention to timing is necessary, even if this means that some groups do not completely resolve their goals. Each step should have an extra layer of responsibility. For example, pairs should generate a list, fours should prioritise or classify the items, and the final grouping should identify common themes that arise, describe the tangential suggestions and agree a summarisation of the work.

Sequenced reports

Reporting back from subgroups to the whole group is a common task in many situations, whether it is in the context of team-building exercises or a conference on personnel management techniques. Adhering to strict rules about timing and asking reporters to use audio-visual aids (e.g. well thought out bullet points in large writing on flipchart paper) can help to avoid the repetitive nature of the process. Setting aside short intervals for reporting with opportunities for interjections, questions and interaction will provide an opportunity for the group to test the validity of the group feedback.

Crossover groups

This is an elegant technique that not only avoids repeated plenary reports but also generates, almost incidentally and therefore with a minimum of fuss, a method of dividing a large group into smaller units in which all of the members meet and work together for a very short period of time. It is also known as the square-root group technique. Participants are divided into groups so that the number in each group is equal to the square root of the total, or as near to it as is feasible. For example, a group of nine would be divided into three triads, and the base group is given a name. Figure 5.2 illustrates a typical labelling convention.

   After a given time period, those individuals who carry the suffix 2 are asked to move to their 'base' table, i.e. A2 goes to table A, B2 goes to table B and C2 goes to table C. This completes the first round. At the next move, group members who carry the suffix 3 move to their 'base' table (A3 moves to table A, B3 to table B and C3 to table C). At each move, the aim is to report the activity of the original group (i.e. A1, B1 and C1) to the new group before comparing notes and re-entering the discussion afresh. This technique is an excellent way of introducing new members to one another, especially on part-time courses where ideas tend to circulate slowly.

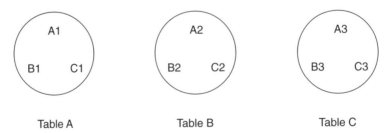

Figure 5.2:   Crossover groups (adapted from Jaques).[8]

Role play

This is one of the most powerful and underused methods in small group work. However, there are good reasons why it is so seldom employed. It is difficult to facilitate, and when poorly structured and guided it can distress participants and severely damage the group. People also shy away either because they have heard about these problems or because they fear the exposure that participating in role play inevitably involves. Thus role-play sessions require experienced facilitators. There are also other drawbacks. Role play is time-consuming, and some people will regard it as frivolous. It requires high levels of motivation, and there is a risk that it may overshadow the need for a parallel grounding in theory and facts.

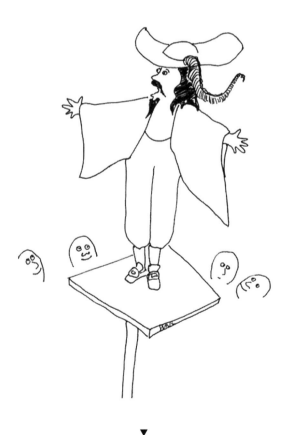

▼
Role play does not mean 'acting'.

At its most basic level, role play involves asking someone to act as if they were an imagined person in a particular situation. van Ments describes asking people to:

> behave exactly as they feel that other person would. As a result of this they, or the rest of the class, or both, will learn something about the person and/or the situation. In essence, each player acts as part of the social environment of the others and provides a framework in which they can test out their repertoire of behaviours or study the interacting behaviour of the group.[9]

Many facets of learning can be explored using the three dimensions of role, situation and learning task (see Table 5.1). However, it must be remembered that the power of the technique (and the reason why it is feared) is that it has the ability to unearth our emotional reactions to situations and the tasks of communicating with other people. This emotional surface is based on our values and attitudes, and the real power of role play (more than any other technique, perhaps) is its ability to generate replicas of our feelings towards people and situations.

The benefits of role play are encapsulated in its immediacy, its ability to 'bring learning to life' and its capacity to make rehearsal safe. It should help participants to:

*   express hidden feelings and discuss sensitive problems
*   understand how others feel and react in different situations
*   observe how some people handle complex, difficult social situations
*   become completely engaged with and captivated by an issue or idea
*   receive immediate and diverse feedback about their performance

Table 5.1:   Three dimensions of role play

Role
Imaginary person: a made-up role which is suggested or described
Real person (inside the group): experiencing another member's perspective and role
Real person (outside the group): imagining an external perspective and role
Self: opportunity to test and display different aspects of perceived role

Situation
Simple (one to one)/complex (group interaction)
Familiar/new
Detailed/broad outline
Short/extended duration

Learning task
First hand (participative)/vicarious (observed)
Skill or technique: opportunity to rehearse and obtain feedback
Sensitisation: opportunity to experience the emotional aspects of other roles
Attitude: opportunity to react and behave using differing attitudinal styles

---

- close the gap between 'theory' and 'practice', and consolidate skill development
- change their attitudes.

van Ments describes a framework that many facilitators use for conducting role play, and his text is one of the key references for those who want to use this method. Figure 5.3 outlines the essential steps.

The commonest way of organising role play is the fish-bowl method. The participants take positions in the centre of the room and the remaining group members sit in a fish-bowl shape around them so that they can closely observe the session. However, there are many variations on the basic process, most of which were developed and described by the Viennese psychiatrist Jacob Moreno in the 1920s.[10] Although he used these methods with patients in therapy and employed the rather worrying term 'psychodrama', they are not in fact difficult to use. They are essentially means to enable participants to explore roles in more depth and from different angles (*see* Table 5.2).

The term 'debriefing', with its military connotations, is perhaps not an ideal one to describe the process that needs to take place after every role-play session. There should be a clear structure to this part of the session, which is best illustrated by describing the following three phases.

- *Describe.* Establish what happened. How did the participants perceive themselves and others? Obtain descriptive accounts of their reactions and emotions.
- *Analyse.* Why did the behaviours occur? Why did particular feelings arise, and what was their impact on the scenario? Establish the cause-and-effect sequences within interactions.
- *Extrapolate.* What does this mean for behaviours and attitudes in the real world? Did the emotional response illustrate attitudes and values which may need to be reconsidered? What could have changed the outcomes? Draw conclusions and lessons to be learned.

Games

Games are 'self-enclosed' rule structures in which the players usually compete in one way or another, and when used for 'educational' or 'personal development' goals they can provide extremely effective simulations of structured environments. The distinction between games, exercises and so-called 'ice-breakers' is developed in Chapter 6 (*see* pp. 105–6). The additional technological dimension of allowing players to interact in 'virtual' environments across any physical distance is expanding the possibilities of this medium, and this area is undoubtedly one of the most interesting interfaces that will develop as 'training' becomes increasingly based on simulation. The Microsoft

Set objectives
Decide how the role play fits into the overall goals (e.g. use the phrase 'by the end of this session, the participants will be able to…')

Setting
Ideally, use a reasonably square-shaped room with a flat floor, and movable furniture to create different situations (e.g. dialogues, small groups or meetings)

Think about the key issues
List the issues that are pertinent to the problem (e.g. a heart surgeon declines a bypass operation to a smoker who has angina; issues to be raised include risks and benefits of the operation, health economics of individual vs. population needs, and ethical considerations)

Decide on structure
Role plays can be descriptive (demonstrate skills and allow others to observe behaviours) or allow rehearsal (by repeated cycles of action and reflection). They can sensitise (enable others to feel what it is like to be in a new role) or facilitate creativity (enable others to behave in new, unfettered ways to gain insight and test reactions). Which structure best fits the learning aims?

Provide material
Write briefs and scenarios or use commercially available packages. Scenarios and role descriptions should not be complex, but they should enable the key issues to surface

Role-play session
Set up role briefings, conduct warm-ups such as a graduated lead in to test roles and participant comfort, running and ending

Debrief
The aim is to allow participants to recover emotionally. Do not underestimate this task. Make sure that participants are able to re-state their identity and real roles before asking them to absorb and analyse the impact of new learning. Pay particular attention to how people 'felt' during the role play. The technique's strength lies in its ability to surface the emotional aspects within interpersonal communication

Follow up
Consider connections to the next activity and evaluate outcomes

Figure 5.3:   Flow chart for use of role play (adapted from van Ments).[9]

Table 5.2: Additional role-play techniques[9]

Role reversal	Protagonists in a debate, for instance, can swap roles or alternative roles can be explored (e.g. teenager plays father, father plays mother and mother plays the teenager). Particularly useful for exploring how individuals (especially adversaries) feel
Role rotation	The lead role (i.e. the role under scrutiny) is moved from one participant to the next, so that all of them have the experience of playing the protagonist
Alter ego	This is a form of role shadowing, where a participant (the alter ego) stands behind the role player and voices the perceived 'thoughts or feelings' of the protagonist, using first-person statements such as 'I was hurt by that comment'. This technique requires experienced role players
Supporter	Role plays can be difficult, and participants often feel 'stuck' when the role play is not going well. The supporter uses the first-person voice again, guides the role player or gives a new direction to the session
Replay	This technique is underused, yet it can provide the necessary rehearsal, confidence and positive feedback that allow tasks such as interpersonal skills to be learned with ease. 'Pause' is another call, and can help to point out a vital feature of the communication process
Fast forward	The role play is going slowly (and missing the main learning opportunities), so the facilitator calls 'cut' and asks the group to assume that X and Y have now happened and proceed from there. This technique requires participants who are very comfortable with the technique, but variations on 'replay', 'pause' and 'fast forward' can be extremely useful techniques if they are used skilfully

games website is an illustration of the scope and extent of 'games' that can be played using a personal computer and a modem.[11] Interactive software can now easily portray a fighter pilot's instruments and the view out of the cockpit and simulate the demands of conducting a flight. Taking part in a group flying exercise is feasible and adds to the challenge. Although such developments are often seen as pure entertainment, there is no doubt that organisations are developing this gaming technology as a means of simulating real experience, both for individual personal development and for problem solving and the development of effective communication skills at a group level.

Used in the more traditional ways, competition within controlled game structures adds considerable momentum to a group, and simulation increases the concentration and attention of individuals, particularly if feedback procedures are integrated into the events. In addition, the vocabulary of the game (members become 'players', their actions and interactions are 'pretend', and any pain or disappointment is entirely transitory – 'it's only a game') provides a secure environment for trial and error.

A detailed description of the games that are used within educational and personal development circles[12–15] is beyond the scope of this book. One that has minimal rules is the 'survival' game in which group members are asked to choose items to help them to handle a crisis. This can be set up as a competitive game, but care needs to be taken to draw out the lessons learned about how the 'problem' was solved (*see* Chapter 14, p. 225) and also how decisions were taken (*see* Chapter 14, p. 238). One example of the many survival scenarios available is provided in Box 5.3.

It is essential to recognise that using a well-chosen game at the correct stage within the lifespan of a group can transform the process and enliven even the most uninspiring group. Many games have a twist in their tail and require either active collaboration or listening skills. The group member who dismisses others, refuses to listen to alternative strategies or declines to share essential pieces of information can be confronted by the results. Such individuals are often startled by the realisation that they have been at the root of their group's failure to succeed, and if handled well this can be a source of great learning.

Although games can take time, require safe and trusting group membership and need careful debriefing, the advantages are numerous (*see* Table 5.4).[16]

Learning sets

This is a fascinating method which involves turning the group concept on its head. The emphasis is not on the group dynamic, but on providing support to the individuals within the group. Learning sets are not transient groups in which individuals can turn up sometimes and miss other meetings. They commonly run for many years, and their members may build up the most supportive relationships they will ever encounter.

What happens in these 'action learning sets' (a term used by one of the key texts)?[17] The concept is simple enough. Participants can work on anything that they wish to bring to the set, and for which they feel the process can be of benefit. The process is the key, and it involves learning from experience, reflection and action. These principles are based on the work of Habermas,[18] Schon[19] and Argyris,[20] and the emphasis that they have given to the feedback loop. Learning sets provide a hothouse for the reflective process, which entails:

- participants reflecting on their experiences and recognising that they have the responsibility for learning
- recognising that reflection is an intentional event
- understanding that reflection is a complex activity in which feelings and cognition are closely interrelated and interactive
- accepting that reflection and learning are cyclical processes.

The key to the process is the structure of a learning set session. For purely practical reasons there are rarely more than half a dozen or so members in a

Box 5.3:   The Simpson Desert: a survival game

The situation

It is approximately 10.00 a.m. in mid-February and you have just crash-landed in the Simpson Desert in Central Australia. The light, twin-engined plane, containing the bodies of the pilot and the co-pilot, has completely burned up, and only the airframe remains. None of the rest of you has been injured.

The pilot was unable to notify anyone of your position before the crash. However, ground sightings taken before you crashed indicated that you are 65 miles off the course that was filed in your flight plan. The pilot had indicated before you crashed that you were approximately 70 miles south-west of a mining camp that is the nearest known habitation.

The immediate area is dominated by sand dunes and, except for the occasional spiniflex, appears to be barren. The last weather report indicated that the temperature would reach 100° – which means that the temperature within 1 foot of the surface will hit 130°. You are dressed in lightweight clothing, short-sleeved shirts, trousers, socks and street shoes. Everyone has a handkerchief. Collectively your pockets contain $2.83 in change, $85 in notes, a packet of cigarettes and a ballpoint pen.

The problem

Before the plane caught fire your group was able to salvage the 15 items listed in Table 5.3. Your task is to rank these items according to their importance to your survival, from 1 (the most important) to 15 (the least important). You may assume that the number of survivors is the same as the number of your team, and that the team has agreed to stick together.

Step 1   Each member of the team is to rank each item individually. Do not discuss the situation or problem until each member has finished their individual ranking. Use the scoring template in Table 5.3.

Step 2   After everyone has finished the individual ranking, rank the 15 items as a team.

Step 3   Compare individual, team and expert scores.*

Step 4   Analyse the problem-solving and decision-making steps that were taken by you and your group.

Step 5   Award praise for the group that survived.

* The expert's listing is provided in Table 5.5 at the end of this chapter.

Table 5.3:   The scoring template for the survival game

Item	Your individual ranking	The team's ranking	Survival expert's ranking	Difference between individual and expert	Difference between team and expert
Flashlight	❏	❏	❏	❏	❏
Penknife	❏	❏	❏	❏	❏
Air map of area	❏	❏	❏	❏	❏
Plastic raincoat	❏	❏	❏	❏	❏
Magnetic compass	❏	❏	❏	❏	❏
First-aid kit	❏	❏	❏	❏	❏
45 calibre pistol (loaded)	❏	❏	❏	❏	❏
Parachute (red and white)	❏	❏	❏	❏	❏
Bottles of salt tablets	❏	❏	❏	❏	❏
1 quart of water per person	❏	❏	❏	❏	❏
A book entitled *Edible Animals of the Desert*	❏	❏	❏	❏	❏
1 pair of sun-glasses per person	❏	❏	❏	❏	❏
2 quarts of vodka	❏	❏	❏	❏	❏
1 topcoat per person	❏	❏	❏	❏	❏
Cosmetic mirror	❏	❏	❏	❏	❏
Total score (the lower the better)	**Score**	**Score**		**Your score**	**Team score**

Table 5.4:   Advantages of games in group work (adapted from Bond)[16]

Increase motivation	Many will associate games with fun and activity, and it is important to preserve this quality even when the games themselves have other aims
Increase involvement	Games are a wonderful way of encouraging the involvement of those who are normally less expressive. The structured rivalry helps to cut across normal dominant influences, and the discussion during the debriefing will be based on activities shared by all of the participants
Transfer responsibility	Forming small competing units provides more opportunity for participants to take responsibility and to experience the nature and role of leadership, without the pressure of performing in a real-life task activity in front of peers
Increase receptiveness	Although it can be difficult to achieve the correct balance, it is vital to keep games light-hearted enough to avoid the generation of anxiety or anger whilst at the same time ensuring that they do not degenerate into frivolity. Participants are more likely to reflect on their behaviours when anxiety levels are low

learning set, because otherwise the group dynamic and timing would become unwieldy. Sets can be organised within organisations, but is it also common to have sets that meet across different organisations and which travel considerable distances. A set would commonly begin by using a round-robin technique. This allows members to 'catch up' with each other after an interval of time, which can vary from a few weeks for sets which provide active support to a few months for sets where members have longer-term goals. The simplest of rounds is to ask 'what's on top?', so that members can spend a minute or two making a statement about what is on their mind. No comments are made or conversations started – the members' task is to listen.

Set meetings are then made up of a collection of individual time slots. As McGill states:

> the essence of a set is to create the atmosphere and use the processes that stimulate learning from action. The actions take place outside the set meeting and often away from other set members. The set provides the focus for the reflective part of the cycle leading to learning from experience and the formation of plans informed by this learning.[21]

Box 5.4 shows the format of a typical learning set.

Providing peer support in a learning set is not as easy as it might sound, and will test the attentiveness of the group. Teasing out pertinent issues or illuminating a key aspect of other people's work requires well-honed listening skills, and members often find that their own abilities as facilitators in other settings develop. Members should ask themselves the following question before making a comment: 'Is what I am about to say going to be helpful?'

Box 5.4:   Format of a typical learning set

Participant 1   *Time allocated 5–10 minutes*
The participant presents their 'project', which can be anything that they want
to work on, to the group. Some projects are problems (working relationships) or
descriptions of tasks and questions about future directions. The key point is that
the member wants to make some progress and would value the group's attention to it. The usual format is to pick up the project for the previous meeting and
use the following framework:

- what I did after the last meeting
- what happened
- what was different
- what I think I learned.

Group members   *Time allocated 20–25 minutes*
The members' task is to help the participant who has just presented his or her
project to explore the issue and discover the options that could be considered.
The intention is not to take the problem away or to solve it, but to provide a
range of views – some that challenge and others that support – thus aiding the
reflective process. There may be some time allowed for the participant to
comment, but it is not a discursive method. The presenter listens to the group's
comments about his or her project, and the session is ended when the facilitator
feels that an action plan has been discussed

Participant 2, etc.
Each participant takes their turn, and the process continues until the cycle has
been completed

Most groups tend to fill the airtime with speech. There is always something
to add, to comment on or to argue against, even if the 'one person speaks' rule
operates. However, it is important to emphasise that silence between comments or questions is acceptable, and is in fact necessary for the presenter to
be able to process the contributions that are made and start the reflective
process. Direct advice is rarely if ever offered. Rather, an open-ended and in-
quisitorial style should be adopted, via questions such as 'What do you think
would happen if ... ?'

It is inevitable that members will get to know each other extremely well,
and that personal details and professional confidences will be shared as participants describe the relationship between work and personal pressures.
Confidentiality is therefore one of the most strongly maintained ground rules
of this method. It must be stressed that the learning set method represents a
very special and intensive use of group work, and should be very well planned
and maintained. There are many features of learning sets that are essential to

understand before embarking on their use, particularly if you are planning to facilitate a set, and further reading is recommended.[19–21]

Brainstorming

Brainstorming (*see* Box 5.5) helps to generate creative ideas and shows how much easier it is to do this when conventional constraints are removed. Brainstorming was developed in the 1930s by Alex Osborn[22] as a way of encouraging groups to generate a range of options and more creative suggestions, and to reduce premature commitment to any one idea because of social pressure.

Box 5.5:   Brainstorming

There are two stages:

* generate ideas
* filter them, preferably against predefined criteria

To obtain the best results, it is important to follow the rules exactly.

1   Arrange two or three hours when you can meet undisturbed
2   Decide on a subject (if you do not have one already) in which change and creativity are important. If one does not come easily to mind, try using the general topic 'ways of improving your teamwork'
3   Start by explaining that the session is going to try brainstorming, which means that everyone is completely free to suggest ideas. Make it clear that all ideas, no matter how absurd or wild, should be contributed, and that there must be no discussion of suggestions at this stage. As soon as one idea has been introduced and recorded, members should go on to the next one
4   Write the rules on a flipchart as a general reminder for the rest of the session
5   When everyone understands the rules, begin the brainstorming session by writing the chosen topic clearly on the flipchart. For example, a useful topic might be 'Ways of improving our teamwork'
6   Brainstorm this topic for about 40 minutes and list (without judgement or discussion) every idea suggested. It is often a good idea to allow individuals to work alone for a few minutes and to list their ideas independently
7   Now divide the team into two subgroups and ask each group to place each idea into one of the following three categories:
   A – important and feasible
   B – possible
   C – worthless
   Allow up to one hour for this phase

continued overleaf

---

8   Ask each group to list all of the 'A' ideas on one sheet, all of the 'B' ideas on a second sheet and all of the 'C' ideas on a third sheet

9   Ask each person to examine both lists of 'A' comments and to choose the two ideas that he or she feels might make the greatest contribution to solving the problem. Each time an idea is chosen, put a tick against it

10   Now take the three ideas with the highest score and ask each subgroup to choose from these the one idea that it feels is the most important. Each subgroup is then asked to produce a written plan for implementing the idea

11   After six weeks, the whole group meets to discuss how well plans are progressing, and to take any necessary action

12   When these first ideas have been successfully implemented, the sub-groups can then move on to the others. Task-oriented subgroups can also be arranged

Social psychologists are beginning to question the value of the technique, and have highlighted three areas of concern, namely 'production blocking', 'free riding' and 'evaluation apprehension'.[23] Others have described the brain-storming process as providing an *illusion* of productivity.[24,25] For instance, it has been shown that brainstorm groups produce fewer ideas than do nominal groups composed of individuals working alone.[23] It is suggested that 'block-ing' may occur because of the rule that only one member may speak at a time, and other members may either forget or feel that their idea has already been contributed, even if it was only partly expressed. Taking a 'free ride' is the equivalent of the broader concept of 'social loafing' in groups – of feeling that one's contribution is not necessary to a successful outcome and therefore letting the group do the work. Despite explicit 'rules' to the contrary, brain-storm participants will inevitably fear that their ideas will be evaluated, even if only at a later stage in the process.[26,27]

Despite the reservations of some critics, brainstorming is still a very widely used technique in education and business, and many would vouch for its effectiveness in raising energy levels to new heights if the method is well conducted.

Reverse brainstorming

In reverse brainstorming, the group is asked to work on exactly the opposite topic to the one they are actually seeking to address. For example, they could use the title 'Ways of *worsening* our teamwork'. The brainstorming session should progress as normal with ideas being noted down in a non-judgemental way. The group should then revisit the list and mark the activities and processes that are currently being undertaken in the workplace. This will then provide an action list of activities that must be stopped for the task (in this case, *improved* teamworking) to occur. It is often both surprising and instructive to identify illogical and destructive activities that are being pursued within the team or organisation. These activities are often suggested merely in jest during a reverse brainstorming session.

Nominal groups

This is a group method that can help to equalise the contribution of all members so that issues of status or assertiveness do not damage the process of generating ideas. A detailed description of this method is provided in Chapter 19. In summary, the technique involves asking individuals to commit ideas to paper (without conferring) before discussing, ranking and agreeing a set of suggestions. This method is considered to be superior to brainstorming as a means of generating a range of new ideas.

Endings

A possible additional stage to those cited by Tuckman[28] is the process that occurs at the end of a series of group meetings. Gorman has suggested the term 'mourning' for this phase.[29] It is certainly true that a palpable sense of grief can exist when a group realises that their collaboration and connectedness have created something unique and of lasting value to their personal development. It is surely correct to recognise this by giving it space and value. Sometimes groups come to a slow end, gradually accepting that the group's function has been achieved, but often (e.g. when a group has formed during an educational course) there is sudden closure, and it is important to provide a structure that matches the climate created.

Speaking rights

One of the most elegant endings is the use of the 'talking stick'. This is based on a Native American tradition of passing round an item which ascribes 'talking rights' to the person who holds it. All of the other participants must remain silent. By explaining these rules and passing the item, the facilitator can invite the members to crystallise their thoughts or comments as a way of providing their final contribution. It seems to help if the item is either unusual or invested with some importance (e.g. a traditional Native American talking stick or a conch as used in Golding's book, *The Lord of the Flies*). This method is particularly appropriate when groups have performed well, and it provides an opportunity for a very positive and cohesive ending.

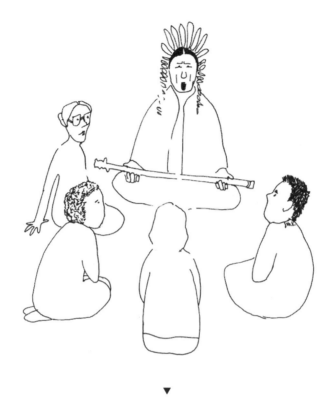

The 'talking stick' ascribes 'talking rights' to the person who holds it.

Personal feedback

Another powerful closure method that is directed more at the individual is to ask each member to write his or her name at the top of a piece of paper. They are then asked to pass it to their immediate neighbour, with the instruction that everyone should write a comment about the individual named on the sheet of paper, usually with the request that the comment should be 'a valued characteristic or behaviour'. Each contribution can be shielded from the next contributor by a request that the paper is folded to cover the previous comments. The process is repeated until the document reaches the named individual again.

Endings can be opportunities for reflection, evaluations, clarification of future actions or summarisation. The golden rule is to plan closures appropriately. If the group has performed very well, provide opportunities for celebration. However, if the group has struggled and battled, allow space for quieter reflection and, where feasible, clarification of how future progress could be made.

References

1   Skinner BF (1976) *About Behaviourism*. Random House, London.

2   Bandura A (1985) *Social Foundations of Thought and Action: A Social Cognitive Theory*. Prentice Hall, New York.

3   Goleman D (1998) *Working with Emotional Intelligence*. Bloomsbury, London.

4   Belbin RM (1981) *Management Teams*. Butterworth Heinemann, Oxford.

5   http://www.teamtechnology.co.uk/home.htm

6   Myers IB (1993) *Gifts Differing*. Consulting Psychologists Press, Palo Alto, CA.

7   Briggs KC and Briggs-Myers I (1998) *Myers-Briggs Type Indicator*. Oxford Psychologists Press, Oxford.

8   Jaques D (1984) *Learning in Groups*. Kogan Page, London.

9   van Ments M (1989) *The Effective Use of Role Play*. Kogan Page, London.

10 Moreno JL (1953) *Who Shall Survive? Foundations of Sociometry, Group Psychotherapy and Sociodrama*. Beacon House, New York.

11 http://www.microsoft.com/games

12 Jones K (1995) *Icebreakers: A Sourcebook of Games, Exercises and Simulations*. Kogan Page, London.

13 Davison A and Gordon P (1978) *Games and Simulations in Action*. The Woburn Press, London.

14 Sugar S (1998) *Games that Teach: Experiential Activities for Reinforcing Training*. Jossey-Bass Publishers, San Francisco, CA.

15 Krohnert G (1992) *100 Training Games*. McGraw-Hill, New York.

16 Bond T (1986) *Games for Social and Life Skills*. Stanley Thornes, Cheltenham.

17 McGill I and Beaty L (1992) *Action Learning: a Guide for Professional, Management and Educational Development*. Kogan Page, London.

18 Habermas J (1974) *Knowledge and Human Interest*. Heinemann, London.

19 Schon DA (1983) *The Reflective Practitioner: How Professionals Think in Action*. Basic Books, New York.

20 Argyris C (1982) *Reasoning, Learning and Action: Individual and Organizational*. Jossey-Bass, San Francisco, CA.

21 McGill I and Beaty L (1992) *Action Learning*. Kogan Page, London.

22 Osborn AF (1957) *Applied Imagination*. Scribner's, New York.

23   Mullen B, Johnson C and Salas E (1991) Productivity loss in brainstorming groups: a meta-analytic interpretation. *Basic Appl Soc Psychol.* **12**: 3–24.

24   Stroebe W and Diehl M (1994) Why groups are less effective than their members: on productivity losses in idea-generating groups. In: W Stroebe and M Hewston (eds) *European Review of Social Psychology.* John Wiley, Chichester.

25   Stroebe W, Diehl M and Abakoumkin G (1992) The illusion of group effectivity. *Person Soc Psychol Bull.* **18**: 643–50.

26   Paulus PB and Dzindolet MT (1993) Social influence processes in group brainstorming. *J Person Soc Psychol.* **64**: 575–86.

27   Levine JM and Moreland RL (1998) Small groups. In: *The Handbook of Social Psychology.* McGraw-Hill, Boston, MA.

28   Tuckman BW (1965) Developmental sequence in small groups. *Psychol Bull.* **63**: 384–99.

29   Gorman P (1998) *Managing Multidisciplinary Teams in the NHS.* Kogan Page, London.

Table 5.5:   The expert's ranking of items for survival

Item	Survival expert's ranking
Flashlight	5
Penknife	6
Air map of area	13
Plastic raincoat	3
Magnetic compass	14
First-aid kit	7
45 calibre pistol (loaded)	12
Parachute (red and white)	1
Bottles of salt tablets	9
1 quart of water per person	2
A book entitled *Edible Animals of the Desert*	11
1 pair of sun-glasses per person	10
2 quarts of vodka	15
1 topcoat per person	8
Cosmetic mirror	4

6

Forming

Piggy: That's why Ralph made a meeting. So we can decide what to do...
Ralph: We'd better all have names, so I'm Ralph.
William Golding, *Lord of the Flies*

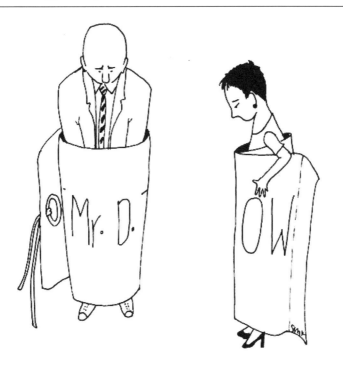

▼

Name labels are an extremely useful way to structure part of the introduction process.

Newly formed groups are often particularly challenging social settings. Individuals react to each other's company in so many diverse ways that it is impossible to predict exactly the interactions that will develop. The process involves different aspects of social integration,[1] of which four varieties have been described.[2]

- *Environmental integration* involves the provision of the physical resources that are needed for groups to form, namely finance, time and people. This is the most basic and traditional level of resources for group formation. These physical requirements are no longer as important as they were in the past. Communication across technological platforms (via email, websites, audio- and video-conferencing) are increasing the temporal and geographical flexibility available to groups (*see* Chapter 12, p. 201).
- *Behavioural integration* is seen when people become dependent on each other to satisfy their needs, which can include social and psychological dimensions. This is the level at which people start to develop group cohesion.
- *Affective integration* is described as the process of 'people starting to develop shared feelings'. This can happen between pairs (chaining) or when a group coalesces around a strong leader (crystallisation).
- *Cognitive integration* is the final stage of group formation, which occurs when people perceive themselves as sharing common and important characteristics. This is when feelings of group 'membership' occur.[3]

The pioneers in the field of social integration were Newcomb[4] and Hyman.[5] Hyman first used the term 'reference groups', which refers to groups to which individuals compare themselves when evaluating their perceived status.

Starting a group

The early stages of group formation are normally characterised by tentative explorations. However, there are methods available to reduce the potential tensions that are created when a group of strangers forms with a view to working together. Some groups are formed for relatively short periods, some are formed in residential or modular courses, while others come together from different departments on a regular basis to solve problems or accomplish defined tasks. The specific context will determine the method that you decide to use, but three key stages have been found to help most groups, namely introductions, ground rules (*see* p. 102) and ice-breaking exercises (*see* p. 105).[6–8]

Introductions

Greeting your colleagues and exchanging names is a very basic step, but even this simple procedure will affect the formation of a group, and if mishandled can unwittingly lead to problems.

Name labels

At conferences it is now customary for name labels to be produced, and it is worth noting their format. Are titles used? Are organisations or occupational roles listed? Would you want to adapt or change the label format for your small group setting? Name labels are an extremely useful way to structure part of the introduction process. Have your own label on display in order to illustrate how it should be completed. Giving everyone a large white sticky label (and instructions to write as clearly as possible the name they wish to be addressed by) has distinct advantages. A less formal and arguably better approach is to pass around a roll of wide masking tape and ask everyone to take a strip. First, it gives the group members something to do, and involves sharing thick black pens perhaps. Secondly, incorrect spellings cannot be blamed on the organiser. Thirdly, the first-name rule (or any alternative convention) is illustrated by default. Finally, names are available immediately for use within the group, and no one has to depend on memory.

Introducing yourself

Participants will feel tentative about a facilitator, whether or not someone else in the organisation has already introduced you. It is good practice to provide the details about yourself that you wish to emphasise. A thumbnail sketch on an overhead projector is one way of giving an outline in a short space of time. Handing out copies of a short CV is another way of respecting the need of the group to know more about you. Another way to build up trust is to offer any details (within reason) that the group wants to know about you. This approach has the advantage of involving the members in an interaction from the outset, and engages that most valuable of human instincts – curiosity!

Structured introductions

The structured introduction can be defined with varying degrees of explicit-ness. The facilitator often leads and the process continues until everyone in the group has introduced themselves. Typically, participants are asked to share some information with the group, such as their role and why they have joined the group. An unexpected and informal element (e.g. 'tell the group something about yourself that we wouldn't normally get to know') can be a useful ice-breaker. Most participants will have encountered this method before, and it has the advantage of being relatively fast, acceptable and fairly non-threatening. There are many ways in which the turn-taking approach can be circumvented or at least modified. Some approaches are outlined in Table 6.1, and these techniques can be easily modified or adapted.[9,10] Whatever way you decide to handle introductions, make sure that the group members have had the opportunity to talk to at least one or two other members before the group convenes formally.

Table 6.1:   Methods of introduction

Activity	Process
Refreshments (e.g. coffee or alternative)	This activity can allow informal discussion between pairs or triads, especially if the facilitator 'works the room', forms connections and introduces new arrivals to established conversations. There is also the added advantage of being able to be flexible about the time to call the group together, which can avoid the common problem of false starts due to late attenders
Sequenced introductions	Members introduce themselves in sequence. This is probably the next most 'natural' method, but be very clear what is required. Use a flipchart to structure contributions, and be aware of the need to give everyone equal time and attention
Paired exchanges	A facilitator asks participants to introduce themselves to each other in pairs, with guidance about time and content. Asking participants to briefly introduce the other member of the pair to the group can extend this process. This approach has many possible variations, has the advantage of not being self-centred, and allows members to test out their listening skills
Rehearsing names	Each participant 'learns' the name of their immediate neighbours on both sides and informs the group. This sequence continues for a full round. Additional variations are possible (e.g. changing positions and immediately repeating the task). Writing names on a flipchart according to seating positions is another commonly used technique for new groups
Collecting 'autographs'	Each participant is asked to write their full name at the head of a piece of paper and then to collect the signature and full name in capitals of every other participant. Although it may seem frivolous, this process has the advantage of speed and physical movement, it can help to loosen things up in the right context, and there are usually some jibes about handwriting and signatures, which act as a useful ice-breaker

Asking for personal details

Beware of using a vague request to start off a round of introductions (e.g. 'Tell us your name and a bit about yourself ...'). For example, if the first participant says, 'Hello. My name is Mrs Lawson. I'm from Bath', then all of the other members are likely to follow suit by making similar minimal statements. However, if the first participant says, 'Hi, my name is Lucy, my interest is riding. I'm here today because my husband has agreed to look after the horses...', and then continues in similar vein for several minutes, the 'introductions' could go on for hours! There may be individuals in the group who have different values and who want to remain more discrete about their personal details (*see* p. 24). Therefore if you decide to use a 'round' of introductions, make sure that you define the task very clearly. A flipchart list or instruction, and an example from you, will help the group members to keep to the brief.

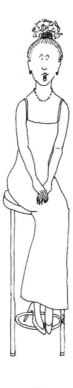

▼

'Hi! My name's Lucy and I'm from Essex.'

Titles

The use of titles, particularly within announced introductions to the entire group, can signal position and associations, give rise to assumptions and prejudice, and may sometimes cause embarrassment. Some facilitators preface their opening statements by using their first name and asking for permission for this to be the norm for the group.

Over the last few decades in developed countries people have generally become more informal in both work and social situations, but the extent of this informality varies between cultures, and between professions and roles in organisations. For example, it is not usually possible to facilitate a primary healthcare team workshop that includes reception staff and clinicians, with the assumption that everyone will be comfortable using first names. Some titles imply hierarchies and role authority, while others designate marital or other status (e.g. religion or armed services).

Ground rules

The best way to get a group to perform effectively is to be extremely explicit about the rules of engagement. These are known as ground rules and, after the introductions, they form the foundations of a successful process.[11] Their purpose is to:

- promote group norms that have the maximum likelihood of creating effective communication
- allow group members to realise and enforce boundaries for their own behaviour and that of others.

Some people can be very insensitive to the views and feelings of others. Rudeness or sexual innuendoes are just some of the inputs that can quickly destroy the group dynamic. Some behaviours are obviously unacceptable, and either the facilitator or the members have to take on the task of challenging and modifying them. This is a difficult process, and is probably best achieved outside the group (*see* Chapter 4, pp. 58–67). However, it is less obvious how to modify the irritations that inevitably occur as a group develops. Someone always turns up late. Another individual may continually huff at various points but never contribute an opinion, suggesting that they are either bored or in disagreement. The facilitator may fail to keep to the agreed times, and although the group work goes well, important decisions and conclusions always seem to be reached in a rush at the end. These behaviours are examples of what can easily become destructive norms.

Establishing ground rules

Unless you are dealing with people who have experience of working in small groups, the participants may not have heard the term 'ground rules' used as a way of establishing expectations of individual interactive settings. In other circumstances where there are organisational 'rules', the team leader may already have a list of rules to govern the group's interactions. In most circumstances, the ground rules should be established (or at least negotiated) by the group itself. They should be clear, simple and capable of being enforced (e.g. 'start and finish on time'). Although it is possible to have rules such as 'kindness', 'politeness' and 'respect for others', these are really examples of a laudable set of *values*, and the boundaries are difficult to gauge. Value-laden rules usually require elaboration (e.g. 'do not interrupt when someone else is talking', 'no personal insults').[11,12]

Asking participants to suggest 'rules' may result in blank looks. The concept may be poorly understood, and it sometimes takes an example or two to set the ball rolling. The facilitator may suggest that one ground rule is 'no smoking during group sessions', or some other suggestion which is unlikely to be challenged. One way of overcoming the block to setting 'rules' is to use buzz groups or brainstorming (*see* p. 89). Experienced facilitators tend to limit the number of rules to around eight or ten, and to have them displayed (e.g. on flipchart paper fixed to the wall). Ground rules can be adapted and changed, and it is good practice to revisit them at each meeting, even if only to check that the members still stand by their previous commitments. Because it is often very difficult to conceive of the types of 'rules' that would be valuable in a group process, one effective technique is to distribute a list of rules (*see* Box 6.1) which can form the basis of either a voting system or a discussion about their priority.

Box 6.1:   A list of possible ground rules for small group work: rules can be adapted and combined as necessary

- ❏   No telephone interruptions (including mobile phones)
- ❏   Start and finish on time
- ❏   Only one person talks at any one time
- ❏   No eating, drinking or smoking during working sessions
- ❏   Everyone is encouraged to contribute
- ❏   The content of sessions is confidential
- ❏   Participation in exercises, tasks and role play is voluntary
- ❏   No lectures
- ❏   Observe agreed timings for exercises
- ❏   Consensus is the aim, but the group will work with majority decisions
- ❏   No sarcasm or insults
- ❏   Use a hand signal to indicate a wish to speak, rather than interrupting (useful in large groups)
- ❏   Allow lateral thinking
- ❏   Facilitators have to abide by the same rules as members
- ❏   No sleeping
- ❏   Other suggestions
- ❏   Other suggestions
- ❏   Other suggestions

Another dimension of ground rules: a group charter

Groups whose main task is educational can perform well if they know the broad aims of the programme and agree to work within explicit guidelines. Groups or teams set up to achieve specific tasks with recognised levels of complexity and fixed deadlines need more than ground rules. Justice has described the process of developing a group charter,[11] which clarifies the responsibilities of the group and removes ambiguities from the decision-making process (*see* Box 6.2). Charters of this nature usually need to be agreed at more than one level in an organisation, and it is essential that they are developed well in advance (e.g. two months) of a group starting to work in earnest.

Box 6.2:   Example of a task group charter

The mission of the University Hospital Task Group on Appointment Bookings is to identify specific strategies to reduce the number of non-arrivals at out-patient appointments

Key problems
- Appointments may be sent to incorrect addresses, as there is no means of checking the patient's current address
- Appointment dates are not negotiated with patients, who may be away or unable to attend for other reasons
- Patients are kept waiting for many months for an assessment of their problem, and the problem may not be causing any further difficulty
- There are no facilities for children in the hospital waiting area (e.g. temporary crèche)

Expected outcomes
- Design method of confirming data about the correct address and the continuing requirement for out-patient appointments (e.g. by evening telephone enquiries)
- Propose a method of offering a range of appointment times (within known clinic slots)
- Research and write a detailed report on the possible introduction of a direct booking system from primary to secondary care
- Facilities for children

Term
The task group will complete its work within nine months of the starting date. Two members will continue to work with the Out-patient Management Group in order to take any agreed recommendation forward

continued opposite

Members

The task group will include the following members:

Alan Brown	Hospital Manager
Surinder Khan	Consultant Neurologist
Sue Hibbs	Finance
Owen Bennet	Information Technology and Communications (Group Leader)
Sally Green	Patient Representative
John Huws	Medical Appointments Office
Facilitator	To be appointed

Professor Araya will serve as the sponsor and confer with the task group leader. She will attend the meetings by request. A review of the work will take place every 3 months, and the final recommendations approved by the Out-patient Management Group will be presented to the Board for decisions regarding implementation

---

A charter is essentially a very clearly worded statement of the purposes of the group, the desired outcomes and the estimated length of time that will be available for the work. During the process of agreeing a charter, it is useful to brainstorm these areas and to list carefully the anticipated problems or obstacles that will need to be tackled in order to address the agreed task (*see* p. 89). The statement should also include the group's leadership and membership, state what happens to the task group at the end of the process, describe the review and reporting arrangements and, depending on the level of detail to be included, indicate the frequency of group meetings and the arrangements regarding costs.

Ice-breakers

The metaphor of breaking ice is a graphic way to convey the purpose of the next stage in the forming process, which is about 'breaking up' the rigidity that most people feel when faced with strangers or a new group, in order to enable easier communication. Good ice-breaker events combine imagination with a reasonable level of challenge. They pose interesting tasks that can be intellectual, practical, creative or managerial in a way that requires communication skills. The aim is to get the group talking and creating solutions, even if this takes place in pairs or triads.

However, this component of small group activity has also acquired a bad name. Many people can recall from painful experience the 'cringe factor' associated with ice-breakers that had more in common with party games than with a considered exercise that enabled better communication.

To avoid the 'cringe factor', it is important to ensure that ice-breakers are *not*:

- extended or contrived introductions (e.g. cushion-throwing exercises)
- simple exchanges of information
- requests to explore feelings and emotions before the group has established sufficient understanding and trust
- potentially embarrassing or demeaning for participants
- contrived, ritualistic or childish.

Exercises, games and simulations

Jones categorised interactive ice-breaking methods into exercises, games and simulations, and his manual provides details of an extensive set of ice-breaking activities.[8] It is important to distinguish between these three terms, because they describe distinct activities that require careful preparation.

Exercises

These are tasks in which individuals (as themselves rather than in other roles) participate to complete a task and resolve a problem or solve a puzzle. Exercises are not in their nature competitive – there is no prize for 'achievement' – and they are the most frequently used type of ice-breaker.

Games

These are 'self-enclosed' rule structures in which players compete in order to win. Competition within controlled game structures adds considerable momentum to a group, and simulation increases the concentration of individuals, particularly if feedback procedures are integrated into the game. Games can be very successful events, but facilitators need to be aware that 'competition' involves winners and losers. Games that require skills that are unevenly distributed among the group may favour a few participants. Mixing participants within smaller subgroups helps to avoid this problem, and it is wise to avoid games that require tasks to be completed by individuals working alone.

Simulation

This is the creation of 'artificial' situations in which activities can be rehearsed and repeated. The technique is not the same as role play (*see* p. 81). Although 'actors' are used in some types of simulation (e.g. simulated patients are used to teach communication skills to clinicians),[13] they are used to recreate the environments in which the participants would expect to function. Participants do not 'mimic' their activities (e.g. achieve decisions, chair a meeting and hold a press conference). Instead, they actually perform these tasks, and are often assessed in the process. Simulations take time to prepare, conduct and debrief, and it would be unusual to use a simulation-type ice-breaker at the start of a group process.

When and how to use ice-breakers

Most facilitators use ice-breakers at the start of a group process. However, there is no need to reserve them for this stage. The communication process can get into difficulties at any time during the life of a group. It is entirely predictable that there will be 'storms' (overt or covert) within groups – energy levels may dwindle, cliques may form and day-dreaming may occur. Ice-breakers can be useful in these circumstances, and can introduce enough creative disturbance to break the patterns and provide fresh ideas.

Therefore one of the most important tasks facing the facilitator is to be clear about the aims of the ice-breaker and how it fits into the overall design of the group process. It is also essential that the participants understand exactly what is required of them. Vague instructions that are only partly comprehended will quickly create chaos and frustration. Ice-breakers, especially the more complex games, need careful explanation and usually require participants' notes. It is important to set aside time for questions before the ice-breaker process begins, in order to ensure that there is agreement and enthusiasm about participation.

The other common cause of failure is to regard an ice-breaker as a self-contained event that requires no debriefing. This tendency to perceive ice-breakers as merely a 'warm-up' routine before the real tasks begin is to deny them their real potential as an introduction to process analysis. Asking participants to share their thoughts and observations (by discussion, brainstorming or 'Post-It' note display) can alert the group to how easy or difficult it is for people to come together and form a group. The time devoted to this type of feedback should be determined by how important it is to get the group off to a good start.

When the authors were researching this book, one of them emailed colleagues working in educational organisations, asking them about their experience of using ice-breakers. Most of the replies indicated how difficult it is to use them successfully. The ease of usage depends on the participants' previous experience and education. Some groups will include individuals who are resistant to engaging in exercises beyond the scope of their day-to-day norms, and in such cases it may be best to use other techniques that achieve some of the same objectives but are less obvious. Boxes 6.3, 6.4 and 6.5 are examples of ice-breakers that have proved useful for many practitioners.

Box 6.3: Ice-breaker – example of an exercise involving negotiation

Half a vote[8]

The aim of this exercise is to agree on topics to put on the agenda of a political organisation. Each participant is given half a vote, but in order to have a valid topic for the agenda, a full vote (or more) is needed. Each individual writes down an important issue for them (e.g. prevention of teenage pregnancy, genetically modified foods) and where they would like this issue debated. By a process of negotiation with others in the group, participants must combine half-votes into a full vote so that the topic can be eligible for an agenda. In other words, pairs must agree on 'issues', and this may require one or both members to change their 'issue'. Individuals do not have to combine votes. However, once pairs have formed they cannot separate, although they can join other pairs and see whether they can combine their votes on a single issue. Any one individual can veto a merger on issues, but once a group consensus has formed the group must always remain together. This exercise needs a reasonable amount of space, as it will generate movement, groupings and regroupings. It is an excellent way of creating purposeful negotiation and a large amount of interaction. Debriefings can focus on the ways in which agreements and negotiations occurred.

Box 6.4: Ice-breaker – an example of a problem-solving game

Paper tubes[16]

The aim of this exercise is to get pairs to work together on a practical task which requires negotiation and collaboration. Pairs are asked to support a tin (e.g. a tin of baked beans) as high as possible above a working surface using three sheets of A4 paper and adhesive tape (three strips of tape, each no more than 3 cm in length). A pair of scissors is also provided. The tin must be supported for at least 10 seconds.

There are a number of possible solutions. Cylinders can be made by rolling the paper along its width or length. The sheets can also be cut lengthways, and a strip cut off one of the pieces. Two long cylinders are then created (by inserting one rolled-up piece of paper inside another) and put together vertically, with the offcut piece acting as a collar (like a double-barrelled gun). The tape needs to be cut lengthways in order to create six strips to support this tubular column. This ambitious solution requires dexterity, patience and the support of a willing collaborator. The debriefing can focus on how the pairs approached the problem and what issues surfaced during the discussion and implementation.

Box 6.5: Ice-breaker – an example of a non-threatening exercise* (contributed by Dr John Plumb, Continuing Medical Education tutor)

Imagine a map

If the group members have come a long way and from all over the place, draw an imaginary map on the floor. Invite people to stand on the area they come from. Individuals will immediately identify with someone who lives relatively near to them. There is usually some amusement when a crowd gathers inside the M25 (the main ring road round London) or two people realise that they share the same postal code. Enterprising foreigners may even climb on the windowsill. Participants will have to move about and come close to each other, and the activity has the advantage of being completely non-threatening. Debriefings can concentrate on the effect that this exercise has had, and the way in which it generates mental models of geography and creates associations and spatial connections between people. The exercise can also be done in stages. For example, go to where you were born, where you live or work now, and where you would like to live.

*Unless you live in Brixton, for example, when everyone else comes from Chelsea. Think through the 'diversity' effect.

Different tasks, different ice-breakers

Some facilitators choose ice-breakers that require behaviours that are beyond the normal experience of group members, while others match tasks to the expected skills. You should always be guided by your aims. Do you want to move individuals out of their usual ways of interacting with people and tasks, so that they can explore new experiences and reactions? This is often referred to as breaking out of the 'comfort zone'. Or do you wish to make a gentler introduction? Here is a brief list of possible outcomes that ice-breakers could help to achieve:

- ask participants simply to talk to one another, reveal their attitudes and understand their perspectives
- get them to co-operate together in order to complete a task
- engage individuals or subgroups in the process of negotiating consensus
- observe behaviours as participants 'compete' within games
- analyse a problem and suggest a range of solutions
- allow the group to display imagination and humour.

Time-limited buzz groups and snowballing techniques (*see* Chapter 5, p. 79) designed to achieve a new mix of participants are less overt ice-breakers, particularly if they focus on tasks that are related but not central to the group's primary aims. For example, a group that wants to solve a bottleneck within their organisation could be asked to work in triads to prepare a presentation from a consumer viewpoint.

The next level of ice-breaking might even take place between formal group events. One course organiser emphasised the potential of allowing participants some free time between sessions and 'plenty of grog'. This method of ice-breaking is often overlooked, or at least comes too late within events (e.g. on the social night on the third and final evening of the course). Never forget the use of breaks in the official task schedule. Something as simple as providing an unusual pack of biscuits at coffee-time can generate a little lightheartedness! An early and long lunch-break with good food that requires some mingling and jostling will allow many participants to start feeling much more at ease.

Toys

A technique that has been described by Justice[11] is the effect of providing toys for the participants. These have been rather grandly described as 'learning aids', and although it is easy to be sceptical or concerned that the toys may act as major distractions, it seems that they put the groups at ease and increase the attention which participants give to tasks. This effect is apparent in both large and smaller groups. The members seem to be more relaxed as they generate ideas whilst 'playing' with malleable balls and investigating the contortions of flexible science-fiction-type figures. The benefits are apparently linked to the technique of allowing 'low cognitive activity while performing higher-order cognitive tasks'. The trick is to find toys that allow people to busy themselves without disturbing others. Examples of such toys include liquid-filled containers of floating particles (snow globes), and adjustable models and figures that can twist and change shape. The toys should not make a noise, be puzzles, or have clockwork mechanisms.

'Initiation rites'

As a general rule, the emotional climate for small group work should be co-operative rather than competitive, and the ethos should be one where individuals are expected to participate rather than to remain passive. Research has shown that harsh or dangerous environments have significant effects on group dynamics.[14] Studies of coal-miners, submariners and astronauts have demonstrated the development of strong leadership, high pressure to conform and immense loyalty and cohesion in the high-pressure work environment.

This in turn helps members of these groups to reduce conflict and to react in a co-ordinated way to problems. Initiation rites and other induction procedures are found within groups that work in situations which require close group cohesion and conformity. For example, coal-miners expose new entrants to frightening and degrading experiences in order to assess how they will respond to the dangers underground, and to demonstrate that safety is a team responsibility.[15]

We are not suggesting that those who work in education, research and management should follow similar initiation rituals. However, it is worth reflecting about the types of induction and group maintenance structures that exist in physically stressful environments, and to consider the parallels with 'team development' or 'away-day' activities that are often held in settings which may appear to have been deliberately chosen to increase members' levels of stress. Group formation is always bound up in one way or another with an appraisal of and adaptation to existing normative behaviours. Junior members or new members of organisations are often asked to undertake the majority of tasks at such events (e.g. to report back at plenaries, prepare a presentation or ensure that a deadline is met). Moreover, group formation takes place at all levels. Eagerness to please, sociability, and reluctance to join in a late-night discussion at the bar are all aspects that are inevitably monitored. Cultures will vary, of course, and what is viewed as necessary in one organisation would induce rejection within others. More senior members of organisations often make judgements about an individual's suitability for acceptance as a full member of the group by observing their performance in such settings.[16]

Box 6.6: Ice-breaker – an example of a more challenging exercise (exercise and theory contributed by Dr Chris Price, Continuing Medical Education tutor)

Juggling

This exercise requires three soft juggling balls for each participant, and enough space and sensitivity in case there are participants with disabilities. The successful execution of three-ball juggling depends upon the mastery of two simple actions, the throw and the catch, performed in a rhythmical and repetitive manner. The aim of the session is to engender a feeling of common achievement and group responsibility for the task.

Decide whether you want to make the objectives explicit before you start. These objectives are that at the end:

- all participants will be laughing
- each participant will be helping a neighbour, even if it is only to pick up dropped balls.

continued overleaf

Theoretical background
This exercise was designed using the learning stimulus–response chaining theory. Gagne described a 'chaining together' of sets of individual 'part-skills' to form a whole task, whereby the individual parts are learned and then sequenced to form the complete skill.[17] The stimulus–response chaining theory is based on the tenet that each component of a complex task is learned individually, and that the retention of the skill is enduring. Gagne recognised the importance of external cues in learning the chaining sequence, and the need for repetition of the learned sequence for reinforcement.

Conclusion

Forming a group does not just happen. As Chapter 10 (*see* p. 159) shows, failure to 'gel' as a group or to set and follow ground rules are two major causes of groups going wrong. The processes of introductions, rule setting and ice-breaking can be condensed or expanded to fit the constraints of your working context, but they should never be omitted. If necessary, it is possible to undertake brief introductions and discuss basic ground rules within the space of a few minutes. However, if a group is meeting together for the first time ahead of a period of concentrated working (e.g. a one-week residential course), then we strongly recommend that you set aside at least two hours to 'form' the group, using some of the techniques outlined above. During this process, personalities will surface and it will become obvious to both the facilitator and the rest of the group which roles the participants are taking on. Some will be focused on the task, while others will be working to maintain the group process. This division of labour is important for the 'performing' stage of the group, and is discussed in detail in the next chapter and in Chapter 8.

References

1   Moreland RL (1987) The formation of small groups. In: C Hendrick (ed) *Review of Personality and Social Psychology*. Sage, Newbury Park, CA.

2   Levine JM and Moreland RL (1998) Small groups. In: *The Handbook of Social Psychology*. McGraw-Hill, Boston, MA.

3   Bar-Tal D (1990) *Group Beliefs*. Springer, New York.

4   Newcomb TM (1952) Attitude development as a function of reference groups: the Bennington study. In: GE Swanson (ed) *Readings in Social Psychology*. Holt, Rinehart and Winston, New York.

5   Hyman HH (1942) The psychology of status. In: *Archives of Psychology*. Columbia University, New York.

6   Jaques D (1984) *Learning in Groups*. Kogan Page, London.

7   Douglas T (1991) *A Handbook of Common Groupwork Problems*. Routledge, London.

8   Jones K (1995) *Icebreakers: A Sourcebook of Games, Exercises and Simulations*. Kogan Page, London.

9   Bourner T, Martin V and Race P (1993) *Workshops that Work: 100 Ideas to Make Your Training More Effective*. McGraw-Hill Book Company, London.

10   Bentley T (1993) *Facilitation: Providing Opportunities for Learning*. McGraw-Hill, London.

11   Justice T and Jamieson DW (1999) *The Facilitators' Fieldbook*. American Management Association Communications, AMA Publications, New York.

12   Weisbord MR and Janoff S (1995) *Future Search: An Action Guide to Finding Common Ground in Organizations and Communities*. Berrett-Koehler Publishers, San Francisco, CA.

13   Kinnersley P and Pill R (1993) Potential of using simulated patients to study the performance of general practitioners. *Br J Gen Pract*. **43**: 297–300.

14   Harrison AA and Connors MM (1984) Groups in exotic environments. In: L Berkowitz (ed) *Advances in Experimental Social Psychology*. Academic Press, Orlando, FL.

15   Vaught C and Smith DL (1980) Incorporation and mechanical solidarity in an underground coal mine. *Soc Work Occup*. **7**: 159–87.

16   Kindred M and Kindred M (1998) *Once Upon a Group: Exercises*. 4M Publications, Southwell.

17   Gagne RM (1985) *The Conditions of Learning and Theory of Instruction* (4e). Holt-Sanders, New York.

—

7

Storming and norming

> *Hell is other people.*
> Jean-Paul Sartre, *In Camera*

In Tuckman's theory of group development,[1] he describes five stages. In the *forming* stage, orientation and exploratory engagements occur. In the *storming* stage, members attempt to change the group to fit their own needs. They suggest ways of working and negotiate positions. It is at this stage that conflict occurs, particularly about roles. During the *norming* stage, the arguments and tensions are reconciled by various mechanisms until behaviours are settled upon that satisfy the groups' aims. In the *performing* stage, members take on roles and work to achieve the agreed tasks. *Adjourning* (ending) describes the withdrawal from these activities. Although alternatives and exceptions have been widely described,[2] as a broad categorisation of the temporal development of groups this approach has proved useful.

Storming

Conflict occurs when people disagree about what they want to achieve by working together. The conflicts that occur in groups are usually complex, and are often based on members' differing beliefs and values, rather than on simple disagreements about shared information. It is essential to understand the nature and origin of conflict, as it can affect the well-being of individuals and influence the performance of the group.

Group dynamics vary in groups of different sizes. The addition of a third person to a dyad changes the dynamic completely, and the original members have to consider how their behaviours will be viewed by the new member. Each additional member increases the number of interactions. Dyads and triads are interesting microcosms of the interactions that occur in larger groups, and some researchers hold that all group processes are accumulations of the dynamics in pairs and triads. Argyle has summarised the literature and notes that a contest for dominance occurs in a triad of three males, and the weakest is relegated, hence the proverb 'three's a crowd'. It is difficult to establish the strength of the evidence for Argyle's assertion that three females tend to work harder than three males to maintain a triad's cohesion.[3] We suggest that this conclusion could betray an element of sex stereotyping.

Overt dominance is not appreciated in any setting, and the collaboration of the weak against the strong is seen both in small group experiments and in real life.[3] As a group increases in size from four to ten or more, the nature of the group interactions changes. It is less easy to participate when size increases, and getting to hold the floor is both a negotiation and a skill, tempered by the anxiety of having an audience to note one's behaviours. In large groups, most members do not normally contribute, and a few members tend to take over most of the decision making. As groups increase in size, even more differentiation occurs, the discussion becomes less inhibited and disagreements are readily voiced, albeit by only a few contributors.

Roles in groups have been defined as 'shared experiences about how a particular person in a group ought to behave'. Storming is essentially a process of testing out role behaviours.[4] Conflict can arise when decisions are being made about roles within the group. Levine has analysed these role issues in depth,[5] and a summary is given below.

Potential role conflicts during the storming process

Role assignment

This is the most common early negotiation. Typical examples include choosing who will perform a task on behalf of the group, such as preparing a report to an external party, or taking the lead on the design and delivery of an event or process. Role assignment can occur at different levels of transparency. More than one person may want a particular role, and competitive bids may be launched, albeit occasionally in ways that are less than obvious (e.g. the ploy of raising doubts about the original decision to do the task).

Role strain

Disagreements may develop about the way in which roles are performed, and this can lead to the recognition that the appointed individual may not have the skills, knowledge or commitment to perform the tasks effectively. This is known as *role strain*. Sometimes new roles are incompatible with those that have already been played. For example, an individual who moves from being a confederate of a group in which it is customary to distrust and complain to being its negotiator for external resources will find it difficult to integrate the two roles, and *inter-role conflict* will occur.

Role ambiguity

Disputes and negotiations arising from the role assignment process will be the main indication that the storming process has started. When individuals start to perform their roles in the group, other tensions will become obvious. There may be uncertainty about the way in which others want them to play the role. For instance, the leadership role can be delivered in many different ways, ranging from authoritarian to consultative approaches (*see* p. 272), and the individual may need to explore styles and test reactions.

Conflict can often be settled by change. Individuals can develop new ways of dealing with colleagues, and when old roles are no longer available or as enjoyable, people either withdraw from groups or establish new behaviours. Like changes made in response to conflict, these adaptations are also part of the storming process and are known as *role innovation* and *transition*, respectively.

Conflict out of diversity

The diversity of membership within a group is one of the main determinants of the way in which it functions. Most recent research in this area has compared groups with differing levels of heterogeneity, and reflects the ethical issues surrounding exclusion from groups on the basis of gender, age, race or religion. Diversity does not improve group dynamics. The greater the differences between group members (whether based on age, gender, culture, professional background or other factors), the less well they will communicate and the less likely they are to develop common understanding – hence there is greater potential for conflict. When this process is left unmanaged, cliques form and groups will become dysfunctional.

However, the flip side of diversity within groups is that, although they have difficult dynamics, they are more likely to generate creative tension. Diverse groups are more flexible, innovate more often, are more likely to detect the need for change, and are more able to adapt to changing environments.[6] There is evidence that the overall negative impact on dynamics can be modified and that groups can learn to manage diversity and make a positive influence on performance more likely.[7] Conflicts can be controlled by educating members about their differences and similarities, and by using techniques that increase tolerance.[8]

The composition of groups or teams is often predetermined. However, there are many opportunities to influence the membership of groups, and although practical, ethical and other problems can arise during selection procedures, it is important to be aware of the potential effects of 'diversity' and homogeneity.

Box 7.1:   Evidence-based healthcare courses in the UK

Two of the authors of this book (Trisha Greenhalgh and Glyn Elwyn) have
organised courses in the UK based on the McMaster model of problem-based
learning and conducted in small groups.[9] The participants come from many
different backgrounds, including nursing, management, professions allied to
medicine, and doctors from a variety of specialties ranging from public health
to psychiatry. How should groups be composed? Should they be composed
around subject areas or specialties, professions or some other category? Should
course organisers make judgements about combinations that would work well?
How diverse should the groups be? Our own research suggests that diverse
groups have much more potential for conflict, but that such groups are also able
to contribute positively to both the educational tasks and the wider process of
professional collaboration.[10]

One way of advancing the argument that fostering diversity can bring
advantages is to list the disadvantages of working within homogenous groups
– of staying within the 'club', so to speak. Individuals with shared values,
backgrounds and beliefs are at considerable risk of having either blind spots
or (worse) narrowly focused tunnel vision. They can share an illusion of
invulnerability and are often oblivious to warning signs, which are either
discounted or ignored. Identical group members often have stereotyped and
usually negative views about outsiders, and may perceive them as stupid,
weak or even evil. The inherent morality implicit in such judgements is not
questioned. Groups of this type are in danger of censoring evidence that
contradicts their world views and suppressing any individual who raises
any doubts about those views in order to create an impression of unanimity
(*see* p. 231).

The main benefit of fostering diversity is the creation of a group culture
in which these types of shortcomings are overcome, at least to some extent.
A spectrum of views will offer marketing advantages (the ability to see products from differing perspectives), cost containment, problem-solving abilities, creativity and system flexibility. As we shall demonstrate in Chapter
15, managing a diverse group is clearly a more challenging task than
managing a group that shares common beliefs and values. This task
therefore requires a better understanding of and motivation to work with
different social, professional and cultural groups. Many commentators
argue that the economic advantages, legal obligations and ethical and social
responsibilities should ensure that group diversity is maximised wherever
this is feasible.[11]

Group norms

Norms are *ideas* that are shared by members of the group about what are acceptable and unacceptable views and behaviours. The early research work on group norms was done by Sherif, who used laboratory settings to observe their development.[12] He placed people in a darkened room and asked them to look at a very small light bulb. Although the bulb was actually stationary, an autokinetic phenomenon (due to eye movement and neural processes) meant that the viewers perceived movement. They were asked to estimate the movement at each exposure. When individuals did this alone, although their initial estimates varied, they quickly settled on a single value (i.e. a norm for them). These norms varied widely between the subjects, suggesting the existence of separate frames of reference.

However, when people were placed together in the darkened room and allowed to communicate, although again their initial estimates varied, as a result of the communication between them the responses soon converged to a single group value. Different groups placed in the same darkened room arrived at completely different values, again confirming that different frames of reference (norms) are established at both individual and group levels. Sherif even manipulated these norms by using 'confederates' to purposely establish high or low values, and confirmed that the artificially created values persisted even when these individuals had been removed from the group. Norms, once established, are persistent.

Sherif found that when a group is forming, many intricate interactions take place which create norms and they affect much of our life, albeit almost imperceptibly. However, we immediately notice when they are broken (e.g. when someone claps at the wrong time in a concert, or when the convention of starting to eat together at a formal meal is ignored, or when swear words are used in contexts that would normally preclude their use). Over time these norms will define the limits of acceptable behaviours and act to control the conduct of group members.[13] Norms are usually implicit in the way that the group is set up and managed. They are also set in more explicit ways by the use of contracts, sanctions and rule setting (*see* Chapter 6, p. 102).

Both existing group members and newcomers to the group will be quick to identify the norms and, depending on their need to achieve safety or conformity, they will adapt to the context. Characteristic ways of speaking and behaving will be observed, adopted or rejected (*see* Box 7.2 for an example from the work context). At the most superficial level, individuals often modify their clothing to fit in with what appears to be regarded as the accepted level of formality. At other levels, attitudes or opinions are monitored and, if not modified, self-presentations are consciously checked.

Box 7.2:   A portfolio support group

Tutors were asked to convene a small group of general practitioners to develop educational portfolios (a collection of accounts and reflections on their learning activities in professional practice). Norms developed very quickly on many dimensions. Dress was 'off-duty' casual, ties were abandoned, bleeps went off, the communication style was informal and based on anecdotes, first names were used, and a jovial, mildly cynical attitude to 'education' developed. The method consisted of discussion, and attempts by the facilitator to encourage the use of a flipchart were declined. Educational jargon was frowned upon (e.g. the term 'needs assessment' was unacceptable), and the attitude to any form of assessment was defensive and reserved.

   This 'norm' was slow to change, and could be contrasted vividly with that of a group of similar professionals who were engaged in a further degree course on medical education. Informality was still a feature of the style, but the normal way of communicating about the 'portfolio' was to reflect seriously on its function as both a lever and a mirror for professional development.

Norms can be measured in several ways. One method is to measure the degree of conformity exhibited by members of the group. Some behaviours pass as normal, whereas others would be considered to display different levels of irregularity, as judged by the reactions they would invoke within the group. Alternatively, group members can be asked to describe the group norms or to relate their reactions to different behaviours by others.

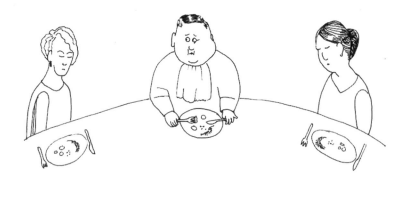

▼

Broken norms: guests start eating before a religious ritual at a formal meal.

Norms, like status systems (*see* p. 25), develop very early within groups and quickly become stable constructs. In other words, early behaviours and appearances rapidly create norms that will remain relatively fixed for the group's duration.[14] Behaviours and attitudes are characteristic of individuals, but they can also be associated with institutions. An organisation will have cultural norms that will be imposed in part by the leadership role within the group or by external stakeholders (*see* Chapter 2, p. 25). Norms can also evolve, particularly when behaviours that are successful (at individual or group levels) are shared and copied. As these behaviours are more regularly exhibited, they are at first anticipated and then eventually become expected conduct.[15] Even when members of groups change, their norms can remain remarkably stable, and when they are positive and strong they can be very important contributors to group performance.[16]

This normalisation process can occur on many different dimensions simultaneously, and Figure 7.1 illustrates the perceived overlaps of members at an early and slightly later stage in a group.[17] This area of agreement can be about group aims, but it can equally represent the norms that members provide for the group, by either informally working together or by a more structured process such as agreeing a group charter or ground rules.

There is always pressure to conform to norms, and continual refusal to do so will lead to rejection by the group. If the deviation concerns a matter of great importance to the group (e.g. if it affects the group's success) then the need to conform will be more urgent. Movement towards the norm occurs for

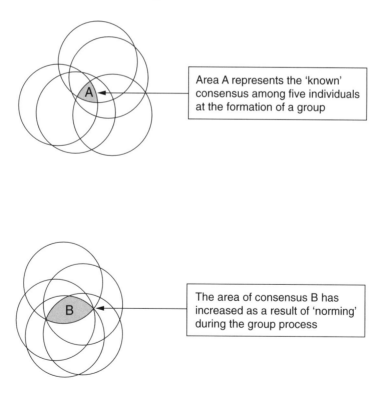

Area A represents the 'known' consensus among five individuals at the formation of a group

The area of consensus B has increased as a result of 'norming' during the group process

Figure 7.1: Increasing agreement and norm setting during a group process.

two main reasons. First, being different 'sticks out' and can make an individual feel silly and isolated. Secondly, majorities are often *perceived* as having valuable information that is likely to be correct. The classic experimental paradigm for studying this issue was developed by Asch.[18] He set up the following task. Individuals had to state publicly, and in a fixed order, which of three comparison lines matched the length of a fourth 'benchmark' line.

The correct answer was obvious, and hardly any errors were made when the judgements were made in isolation. However, Asch then put naive subjects in a group of confederates, who were instructed to agree on an incorrect response. Only 25% of the naive respondents remained independent and adhered to the correct judgement when they were exposed to the publicly expressed viewpoints. In other words, 75% of them conformed to the majority view. This may explain why groups often make major errors in decision making, and are unprepared to change their views even in the face of overwhelming factual data.

However, there are times when an individual deviates from group norms and the interactions that occur follow recognised patterns. Surprise is usually expressed with non-verbal language or laughter. There are three possible outcomes – ideas or behaviours are either rejected, ignored, or occasionally recognised as a possible innovation. Deviant behaviour that has the potential for being rewarded with success for the group is more likely to be explored, and in some fields (e.g. science, art and fashion), deviation is, to some extent at least, encouraged and earns 'idiosyncrasy credit'. Deviant behaviour is much more likely to lead to change if two members uphold the ideas. Unanimous minorities who have conviction are the most potent agents of change within groups.[19]

Group structure and status systems

The norms that come into existence in a group are part of its structure, and although they can vary enormously between examples, research in this field has demonstrated that these structures develop quickly at the inception and formation of the interactions, but subsequently change very slowly. Subsequent attempts at reorganisation evoke anxiety and are likely to encounter resistance.[5]

Status systems exist within groups and represent how power is distributed between the members. Individuals with higher status have been observed to maintain longer eye contact and more upright posture. Verbal behaviour is also a marker of status. Those who are perceived to have high status will be 'spoken to' more often, but they also speak more loudly, and are more likely to interrupt and criticise.[20] It seems that status is ascribed, not earned. This view has been proposed because status systems have been noted to develop within minutes of some groups forming, which conflicts with the suggestion that status is a reward for contributions made to the group process.

Two theories have been proposed to account for the development of status that may be lower or higher than the individual actually deserves.[21] The theory of 'expectation states' argues that status is ascribed on the probability that individuals will contribute to the group's aims, and that it is calculated on the basis of disclosures and statements made about previous experience or achievements. Status ascribed in this way is more easily lost than gained. In other words, individuals who are assigned low status will have difficulty in gaining ground within the group structure.

The second group of theorists propose that strengths and positions are gauged by appearance and behaviours, including size, facial features, body language and verbal turn-taking.[22] Those who stand out as having low or high status according to these criteria are assigned status immediately. Others must engage in 'contests' which, although they can be covert (e.g. refusal to share a quip, or speaking out before others have completely finished their turn), are nevertheless part of the process that defines the structure and norms within the group.

More recent research suggests that these two theories should be integrated, and that the attribution of status depends on both ability and perceived strengths, and that claims and counter-claims for positions depend on a mixture of factors which will be conveyed by both individual and group behaviours. However, the evidence clearly indicates that these positional norms are slow to change. People with high status tend to enjoy being in a group more, and it may not be in their interest to make changes. They also receive more positive evaluations within the group, which in turn serves to consolidate the group structure. Efforts by individuals of lower status to introduce changes are made more difficult.

Taking part in small group work: maintenance and task roles

Whenever a group comes together, its individual members to varying extents take on two key roles. First, they contribute to the main objective of the group (task achievement) and secondly they contribute to the cohesion of the group (its maintenance). These two activities – group maintenance and task achievement – are usually interwoven, but some individuals are naturally better at one activity or the other. However, it is possible to adapt behaviours according to need. Good facilitators spot the gaps and make sure that participants contribute to make good the deficits.

Maintenance and task roles are important because:

- individuals may have to *take on* roles in order to make the group function
- an individual can learn to extend their repertoire of roles and thereby increase the effectiveness of group work.

The development of group roles has been measured in many ways, including questioning and observational techniques.[23] It has been found that maintenance roles (*see* Table 7.1) are slower to develop within groups because most individuals first take on task-related activities (*see* Table 7.2). Speculation exists as to whether roles are developed according to the needs of the group, or whether they are imported from previous contexts. The consensus seems to be that individuals who succeed at a role within one group can repeat the role within another and that previous group achievement can serve as a model for other groups and the range of roles required.[24] Having clearly defined roles contributes to better task performance and group dynamics.[5]

These two facets of groups – task achievement and group maintenance – define the two motivations for joining any small group. Although some social groups (e.g. circles of friends) have very minimal formal tasks, some kind

Table 7.1:   Maintenance roles

The supporter	This role provides the warmth and well-being which is part of the group's support framework (e.g. verbal support for a contribution, such as 'Yes, that's a good suggestion', or non-verbal gestures, such as nodding and smiling. Many members who say very little are actually extremely important supporters merely on account of the contributions they make via their non-verbal language
The joker	Many groups have survived because of intermittent injections of light relief. Letting off steam in this way is important when the task has become an all-consuming objective. However, humour can also be destructive and counter-productive if it trivialises the task or undermines contributions. However, humour that is insightful and well meant helps to maintain a positive group dynamic
Experience sharer	When a member of the group shares a personal experience that is both relevant and helpful, it often has the effect of enabling members to understand the issues on a deeper, more intimate level. These types of contribution can also help professional groups to avoid the tendency to become bound by formality
Process observer	When a group has a problem or grows tired, the *process observer* stands back and says 'This is what I think has happened here...', and goes on to provide a 'meta-assessment' of the group process. This role helps the members to evaluate the group's development and to share ideas about the next steps

Table 7.2:   Task roles

The initiator	This is the person who gets the ball rolling. This could be the nominated leader, but not necessarily. The initiator provides impetus, perhaps at different stages, and may well be able to change direction or even modify the task
The clarifier	This role reformulates contributions, teases out their precise meaning and identifies how different contributions relate to one another
The information provider	This role either has the information to hand or is prepared to obtain and contribute information as and when it is required
The questioner	This role asks basic or fundamental questions about the task, but also steps back from the action and challenges the group about the assumptions that may underlie the process
The summariser	This role pulls together the various contributions into a conclusive whole. It does not add anything new to the group's thinking, but checks what has been achieved and what still remains to be done. This role is particularly important when a group gets stuck and lacks direction

of leisure activity is normally constructed to provide a vehicle for the group interaction. The successful integration of these two roles by group members, and the balance that is struck between social enjoyment and the attention given to completing the task, are critical to achieving successful outcomes. Task and maintenance roles are discussed further in Chapter 8 (*see* Tables 8.3 and 8.4 on p. 137).

After the storm...

It is never very clear when the 'norming' and 'storming' processes (which are clearly interrelated) are abating. In fact, after an initial rapid normalisation phase, the norming process is sustained as new influences impinge on the group. It is important to beware of underestimating the need to explore these early stages of group evolution, particularly if the group members face an extended period of time together. If you are starting off with individuals from diverse backgrounds or work cultures, make sure that you have carefully addressed the presumed acceptance of norms, and find out whether there is a storm brewing. It is better to release the energy of a potential conflict at an early stage than to risk an explosion at a more critical stage (e.g. when the group is actively performing its task or approaching a time-critical or public presentation of achievements).

References

1   Tuckman BW (1965) Developmental sequence in small groups. *Psychol Bull.* **63**: 384–99.

2   McCollom M (1990) Re-evaluating group development: a critique of familiar models. In: J Gillette and M McCollom (eds) *Groups in Context: a New Perspective on Group Dynamics*. Addison-Wesley, Reading, MA.

3   Argyle M (1994) *The Psychology of Interpersonal Behaviour* (5e). Penguin, Harmondsworth.

4   Fisher CD and Gitleson R (1983) A meta-analysis of the correlates of role conflict and ambiguity. *J Appl Psychol.* **68**: 320–33.

5   Levine JM and Moreland RL (1998) Small groups. In: *The Handbook of Social Psychology*. McGraw-Hill, Boston, MA.

6   Milliken FJ and Martins LL (1996) Searching for common threads: understanding the multiple effects of diversity in organisational groups. *Acad Manag Rev.* **21**: 402–33.

7   Watson WE, Kumar K and Michaelsen LK (1993) Cultural diversity's impact on interaction process and performance: comparing homogenous and diverse group tasks. *Acad Manag J.* **36**: 590–602.

8   Moreland RL, Levine JM and Wingert ML (1996) Creating the ideal group: composition effects at work. In: E Witte and J Davis (eds) *Understanding Group Behaviour. Small Group Processes and Interpersonal Relations*. Erlbaum, Hillsdale, NJ.

9   Sackett D, Scott Richardson W, Rosenberg W and Haynes R (1997) *Evidence Based Medicine. How to Practise and Teach EBM*. Churchill Livingstone, New York.

10 Elwyn G, Rosenberg W, Edwards A *et al.* (2000) Diaries of evidence-based tutors: beyond 'numbers needed to teach'... *J Eval Clin Prac.* (In press.)

11 Schneider SC and Barsoux J-L (1997) *Managing Across Cultures*. Prentice Hall, London.

12 Sherif M (1936) *The Psychology of Group Norms*. Harper and Row, New York.

13 Myers DG (1993) *Social Psychology* (3e). McGraw-Hill, New York.

14 Feldman DC (1984) The development and enforcement of group norms. *Acad Manag Rev.* **9**: 47–53.

15 Opp KD (1982) The evolutionary emergence of norms. *Br J Soc Psychol.* **21**: 139–49.

16 Argote L (1989) Agreement about norms and work unit effectiveness: evidence from the field. *Basic Appl Soc Psychol.* **10**: 131–40.

17 Douglas T (1991) *A Handbook of Common Groupwork Problems*. Routledge, London.

18 Asch SE (1955) Opinions and social pressure. *Sci Am.* **193**: 31–5.

19   Moscovici S (1980) Toward a theory of conversion behaviour. *Adv Exp Soc Psychol.* **13**: 209–39.

20   Skevotetz J (1988) Models of participation in status-differentiated groups. *Soc Psychol Quart.* **51**: 43–57.

21   Berger J, Rosenholtz SJ and Zelditch M (1980) Status organizing processes. *Annu Rev Sociol.* **6**: 479–508.

22   Mazur A (1985) A biosocial model of status in face-to-face groups. *Soc Forces.* **64**: 377–402.

23   Rose J (1994) Communication challenges and role functions of performing groups. *Small Group Res.* **25**: 411–32.

24   Hare AP (1952) Types of roles in small groups: a bit of history and a current perspective. *Small Group Res.* **25**: 433–48.

8

Performing

It might seem logical that once a group has formed (i.e. broken the ice and completed introductions), stormed (i.e. allocated and tested task and maintenance roles) and normed (i.e. members have adapted and accommodated to each other), it could then simply get on with its business. However, the process of performing (i.e. using the group process to achieve the group's agreed objectives) is never straightforward. In particular, there needs to be a constant cycle of observation, reflection and intervention in order to:

* avoid excessive adherence to group norms
* identify and manage conflict

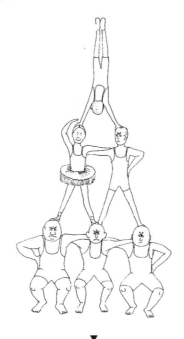

▼
Performing.

- probe problems and review agendas
- ensure that everyone in the group pulls their weight and that everyone's skills are used appropriately
- ensure that the task is achieved, while at the same time an effective and sustainable group process is generated, so that members can continue to work together effectively.

During the norming phase (*see* Chapter 7, p. 122), the members of the group acknowledge shared interests and adopt shared perspectives and patterns of thought. This process has been called 'cognitive tuning', and it undoubtedly strengthens the overall resolve of the group to achieve the task.[1] However, the social conformity required for cognitive tuning can also swamp important minority views and innovative approaches, and overlook data that could be of vital importance.[2] Because of this tendency, methods need to be devised to control the norming process and prevent premature consensus seeking.

On the other hand, when groups are storming, the opposite process occurs and individuals are 'tuning their own interests'.[1] The judgement as to what is an innovative minority contribution rather than a self-seeking strategic intervention is one of the most difficult to make with certainty. The phenomenon of 'social loafing', where some members take a free ride on the back of other contributions, has been explored in detail in the experimental setting.[3] Groups that perform well have managed to overcome the conflict between common and individual interests, and have developed strategies that avoid the all-too-common finding that the bulk of the work is done by one or two participants.

Schein described the methods used to support group work as 'process consultation',[4] and his work was later developed by Reddy.[5] This chapter draws on their descriptions of the methods that they found useful.

Process consultation: maintaining the effectiveness of the group process

Reddy defined process consultation as:

the reasoned and intentional interventions by the consultant [facilitator] into the ongoing events and dynamics of a group with the purpose of helping that group effectively attain its agreed-upon objectives.[5]

Process consultation has a similar aim to the 'time-out' technique described in Chapter 4 (*see* p. 58), but it is a more structured and formal approach with greater emphasis on helping the group to modify its own processes. The purpose of the method is to increase the ability of the group to consider the 'what and how' of the tasks that they face. Most process consultation interventions will be directed to the whole group, but occasionally subgroups or individuals may need individual attention. Interventions should ensure that the group, and not just a few motivated individuals, has:

- taken on the responsibility and ownership of the tasks
- shared information openly and in sufficient detail for effective decision making to proceed
- probed and analysed problems in sufficient depth to allow a range of possible solutions to be considered.

The intensity, timing and design of process consultation interventions will vary according to the intended purpose of the exercise. Table 8.1 lists the methods most commonly used to address group performance. Reddy's iceberg

Table 8.1:   Performance reviews

Agenda review
It is common for groups to agree agendas at the start of a task but then to slowly realise that their ideas have changed. What seemed like a good idea is no longer inspiring. It is also possible that a suggestion was taken up by the group merely because everyone assumed that the group agreed. Silence does not automatically mean affirmation, and this false consensus has been described as the Abilene paradox.[6] It is vital therefore periodically to check that the group is still happy with the direction of travel, and remains committed to it

Observational feedback
This intervention involves describing the recently witnessed process in terms of individual behaviour and group dynamic and emotional climate. For example, the statement, 'three members have spent an hour enthusiastically discussing and agreeing that the team will change its marketing strategy' will, in most circumstances, be enough of a stimulus for reflection about the hidden emotional and behavioural agendas

Reconstruction
This requires an accurate historical analysis of the group process and discussion about possible modifications that could have changed the existing outcomes. Some groups may be capable of simulating dynamics at previous points in time and re-entering the process to re-experience different approaches

Projection
This is probably one of the most difficult reviews to conduct successfully, and it requires high levels of confidence and trust among the group members. The group is asked to simulate one or more 'projections' of the process that has been evolving. The use of 'fast-forward' techniques can be useful here. For example, participants can be asked to imagine the 'what' and the 'how' of the group process at an agreed point in time. The power of the technique lies in allowing different group dynamics to be tested. For example, some people who are normally reserved can be asked to play a dominant role so that the effect on the process can be witnessed. The method is an adaptation of 'simulation' and it is a powerful way of improving group performance

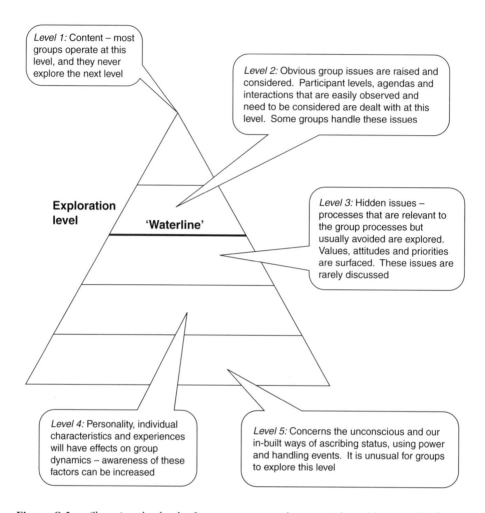

Figure 8.1:   Changing the depth of group process exploration (adapted from Reddy).[5]

metaphor (*see* Figure 8.1) has been adapted to illustrate the 'exploration level' of process awareness that exists in every group. We have probably all been in groups where most of the members seem to be unaware of anything apart from the most tangible aspects of task content. Process consultation, like most facilitation methods, allows deeper exploration of the hidden processes, conflicts and undercurrents, even at times allowing glimpses of the sharks and other monsters that lurk within individual characteristics. Techniques that delve into personality issues, such as the Myers-Briggs Type Inventory (*see* Chapter 5, p. 76) are extremely powerful tools that can help to plumb the lower depths.

Performance reviews

Analysis of process cannot be carried out unless the full range of facilitation skills is used (e.g. actively listening, clarifying, summarising and testing consensus as the group functions) (*see* Chapter 4, p. 57). In addition to these generic methods, specific performance review methods, as listed in Table 8.1, can be introduced.

Encouraging participation

Group performance will be enhanced if there is an ethos of equal participation and contribution. This does not necessarily mean that all members have to talk and make suggestions. Participation by supporting others, nodding, affirming and being prepared to take on tasks is as important as being overtly involved. Non-participation becomes obvious very quickly (*see* Chapter 4, p. 58). Gaze is diverted away when responses are required, the shoulders are shrugged and the non-participating member will ask tangential questions, or reopen issues that have already apparently been resolved. These are warning signals and deserve attention.

Table 8.2 outlines some techniques that can improve the equity of participation within groups. Some of these approaches carry higher risks than others.

Table 8.2:   Increasing participation

Divide and allocate
There are two main strategies. Putting non-participatory members together can have the effect of allowing problems to surface. They share reasons for disgruntlement and feel more confident to share them with the wider group. Putting non-participants and active contributors together often gives the timid participant a voice, but it also runs the risk of repeating the patterns of the large group. An extension of this technique is to 'snowball' (*see* Chapter 5, p. 79) – that is, to join small groups together, pairs forming quartets, etc.

Introduce an 'ice-breaker', game or simulation
These techniques should not be reserved for the early stages of the group process. Structured exercises which involve problem solving, games which introduce competition, and simulations which involve all of the group can increase energy and participation levels if introduced skilfully (*see* Chapter 5, p. 83 and Chapter 6, p. 105)

Sequenced turns
Using 'rounds' where everyone participates in turn is an effective method of making sure that everyone contributes, and indeed feels obliged to take part. The disadvantages stem from the tendency of the round to become tedious, especially if some members hold the floor extensively. The method works very well when the group is addressing an issue of importance, where it is vital to hear every view, even if they are all affirmatory

continued overleaf

Participation hill

A very effective way of raising awareness about participation is to ask participants to position themselves on the 'hill of influence'.[7] Using a bold colour,
draw three concentric circles on a large piece of flipchart paper and explain
that these are contour lines that delineate a hill. The inner circle represents
the summit of the hill and the position of greatest influence on the group
process. Individuals are asked to write their name on a small adhesive note
and place it at a point within the three circles that represents their perceived
level of participation.

When all of the group members have positioned their notes, a discussion
about the ascribed positions is almost bound to occur. For example, there will
be differences between self- and group-ascribed positions. Research on group
process indicates that the most effective group performance occurs when
participation levels are balanced, as illustrated in Figure 8.2. The advantage

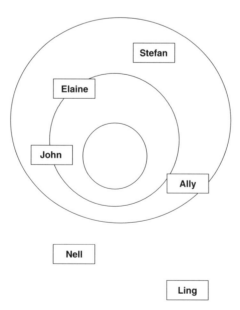

Figure 8.2:   Participation hill, showing member participation (with outliers).

of this technique is that it externalises views and opinions about self-perceived participation levels. By repeating the task at intervals during the group process, either half-way through or at the end of a particular phase of work, the group process is both made explicit and recorded for future reflection by the group. The performance is made part of the group memory.

Group memory

The communication process in a small group is necessarily multidimensional. Although it is possible to discern agreements and decisions, it is also extremely likely that different members of a group will have drawn different conclusions and come away with different understandings during group interactions. It is important therefore that a system of recording and substantiating the group's memory is in place, especially if the task is complex and the work is to be sustained over many group sessions. Two steps are essential to achieve this objective. First, a recorder or scribe should be appointed, and secondly, a way of transcribing the recorder's notes into a format that is approved by the group as a whole should be agreed upon.

Appointing a recorder is not a straightforward task, and it is very difficult to know who has the necessary skills in a new group. This is best explained before the task is assigned or a volunteer steps forward. The individual must be prepared to capture the group's views, not their own interpretation of the events, and must therefore consult regularly with the group in order to agree how their decisions are to be recorded. They must also be familiar with the content of the discussions and language used within the group. Novices, new members or clerical members are often asked to act as recorders and then struggle to capture the exact meaning of the discussions. They have difficulty in understanding and therefore summarising the interactions accurately. The role can be rotated, but make sure that the recorders can work at speed, are adept at consulting and are able to be flexible about the way in which events are recorded. It has been shown that groups which have a competent recording capacity at least double their speed and output.

How to be a group recorder

- Record actual words and statements – don't interpret.
- Become invisible and avoid becoming a co-facilitator.
- Write in a large hand (letters roughly 10 cm in size, e.g. thumb-height letters).
- Be quick, and don't worry or ask about spelling.
- Use brief clarifying questions, but sparingly.

- Use abbreviations and jargon which are understood by the group.
- Date and label flipcharts if you intend to use them in the future.
- Use simple graphics and a maximum of three colours.

There are many ways in which the record of the group's transactions can be displayed, and it is important that the notes are shared and agreed before they are accepted as visual cues to enable the group to look back and reflect on their process. The time-honoured approach is to attach flipchart paper to walls or other convenient surfaces, and this has the advantages of immediacy, adaptability and flexibility. Other methods, such as circulating copies of minutes or projecting notes from a laptop computer, may introduce too much formality and convey the impression (sometimes correctly) of ownership and manipulation by the recorder or reporter.

Storyboard

The work involved in displaying data, especially how complicated systems are broken down into their component parts, often reveals new information and innovative ideas about how things could be changed and improved. This sequential laying out of actions and stages is essentially a form of storyboarding, a technique borrowed from the film world, in which sketches of scenes guide the production tasks and provide a flexible shorthand for making changes to the flow and construction of the visual end-product. Similarly, storyboarding can provide a framework for the same type of creative planning for small groups, where it is also known as 'displayed thinking'.

Detailed descriptions can be found elsewhere,[8,9] but, in summary, different sized cards are provided on which members either draw images or write short phrases to convey 'ideas, steps or stages that would accomplish our goal'. These are then assembled on a board and the mobility of the cards enables new configurations to be proposed. The group can then refine the stages in more detail, or cluster cards together to create new pathways before transferring the agreed 'storyboard' to a more constricting medium such as a flipchart.

Many sophisticated card systems with hierarchical sizes to determine layers of tasks are now available. There are specialised kits available, such as reusable blank hexagons that fit together to form geometrical shapes as a way of modelling complex organisational and inter-agency relationships using a total systems approach.[10] They are all essentially ways of getting ideas into explicit tangible formats, so that groups can manipulate the data with more ease.

Task and maintenance behaviours, and how to spot them

Effective and sustained group performance will depend on balanced participation, open communication about differences and conflicts, and attention to the two types of behaviour that group members must employ, namely task achievement and group maintenance.[11] Too much emphasis on task at the expense of maintaining the group, or vice versa, will – if left unchecked – cause dissent and low morale. Details of these roles can be found in Chapter 7 (*see* pp. 124–5), but it is important to know how to check that they are being actively employed by the group members. Tables 8.3 and 8.4 list the types of comments and phrases that illustrate contributions to task and maintenance roles, respectively.

Table 8.3: Examples of task role behaviours

Task	Example
Proposing	'Let's try to...' or 'I think we should...'
Testing consensus	'Does everyone agree that we could...?'
Consolidating	'I agree with that, and it would do...'
Clarifying	'Do you mean that if we took that approach...?'
Questioning	'Do you really think that we could hope for that outcome...?'
Contradicting	'I don't agree. That could cause all sorts of problems...'

Table 8.4: Examples of maintenance role behaviours

Maintenance	Example
Motivating	'We're doing very well, actually. Better than I thought...'
Lightening	'We're in danger of missing lunch here, let's get our priorities right...'
Observing	'We've got stuck on this one. Maybe it's time to take a break?'
Praise	'Jack really hit the nail on the head with that point.'

Techniques for resolving conflict

Groups will always experience conflict. It is the way in which these conflicts surface and are handled and resolved that will lead to either success or failure.

1 Acknowledge that conflict exists

The group has to be brave enough to pinpoint the issue and then tease out exactly where the disagreement lies. The disagreement may be fundamental or it may be about one small component (e.g. cost) rather than, for example, the principle of purchasing a new alarm system for the hospital. Listing the exact areas on a flipchart helps to distance people from their emotional reactions and assumptions.

2 Recognise potential benefits from the conflict situation

Some experienced facilitators actually enjoy handling conflict. Such situations release energy and real feelings, and if handled positively they can lead to creative solutions. If a group seems anxious about facing the 'dark' side of some problems, it may be worth asking them to reflect in general terms on the potential beneficial outcomes that may result from an overt conflict. This can be done by discussion, buzz groups or brainstorming.

The group may arrive at something similar to the following list of benefits:[12]

- increasing understanding and respect
- exchange of views and attitudes
- feelings surfacing
- expression of energy and motivation
- self-awareness
- creativity
- novel approaches
- full extent of diversity revealed
- opportunities for change.

As we all know, conflict also leads to many problems. The above list is not an attempt to deny the potentially harmful effects of conflict, but a way of helping a group to face such problems in a positive and purposeful way.

3 Consider the options for handling conflict

The assertive – co-operative grid (*see* Figure 8.3) illustrates graphically that there are a number of ways in which groups can choose to handle conflict. Drawing attention to these options can help individuals in a group to recognise where their behaviour lies, and can lead to substantial shifts in the way in which group members approach a resolution.[8]

4 Distinguish between interests and positions

If the group is prepared to do this, another useful exercise is to ask the participants to differentiate between 'interests' and 'positions', between the 'what' and 'why'. For example, a chief executive of a company may wish to set up an appraisal system for all of the staff, but finds that there is resistance from all levels. What he wants to do is to *appraise staff in order to develop and reward good performance*. No one in the company has any real difficulty with the 'what'.

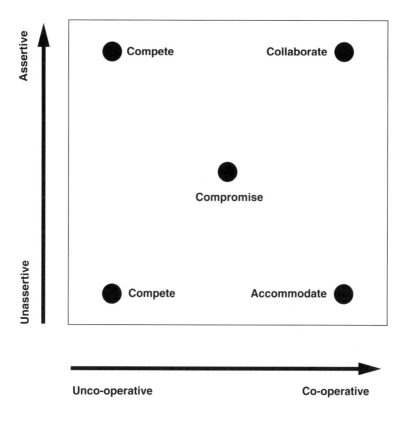

Figure 8.3: Assertiveness vs. co-operative conflict resolution.

However they do worry about his 'interest' in the proposed system. They may mistakenly assume that he intends to rank their performance in order to identify candidates for redundancy.

Box 8.1 summarises an exercise that can be used to elucidate the differences between 'interests' and 'positions'. It is likely that this method will eventually uncover some areas where the parties may have certain interests in common. If not, at least they will probably understand *why* they disagree, and will be aware of each other's basic assumptions.

Box 8.1: Expressing 'interests' and 'positions'

- Two participants stand facing each other. One party is asked to state their positions.
- The opposing participant asks 'Why is it important to you?'
- Responses are recorded.
- This question is repeated until the answers are exhausted.
- The process is reversed, and the group discusses the insights that are obtained by separating out the interests and positions.

5 *Try using 'and' instead of 'or'*

Commonly known as 'the *and* test', it often comes as a complete surprise to people that conflict was not actually necessary. It is entirely possible (in fact, common) for people to draw battle lines because they have got into the 'either/or' fixation. If you run the two positions together using 'and' instead of 'or' in the same sentence, the realisation that the concepts are not mutually exclusive can lead almost magically to new solutions. At the very least it offers a proposition that can be brainstormed for potential compromises.

Box 8.2:   Problem- or topic-based curriculum?

A group of educators in paediatric nursing are arguing about a new curriculum for first-year student nurses. The two most senior members feel that the previous year's timetable should be followed again, with topic-based sessions such as 'care of the asthmatic child', 'nutritional needs of the newly weaned infant', and so on. However, two younger members have had a taste of problem-based learning methods, with sessions covering whatever clinical problems happen to arise on the wards.

After a heated discussion, the group comes to realise that both of these approaches are possible, so long as key topics are identified sufficiently well in advance for the students to prepare relevant case presentations based on their experience with patients.

---

6 *Acknowledge and face up to 'cultural' differences*

Conflict often has roots in deeply held values and attitudes, which is why some disputes are apparently impossible to resolve by focusing on the facts. For example, consider the classic cultural divide that Justice describes when efforts are made to resolve conflict between groups of trade-union workers and senior managers.[8] Box 8.3 illustrates the separate cultural territories that, by virtue of their interests and values, they inhabit. Resolving industrial

---

Box 8.3:   Cultural and value-based territories

Trade-union values	*Management values*
• Mutual protection	• Performance and competition
• Solidarity and brotherhood	• Competition and ascendancy
• Equality	• Pecking orders
• Democratic process for decision making	• Rational analytical decision-making process
• Rules based on precedent and history	• Pragmatism
• Challenge the company ethos	• Shareholder value and profit

---

disputes involves communication between these contrasting value systems. Cultural differences are discussed further in Chapter 15.

Reverse argument postions

The statement 'before you argue with me, argue for me' is one of the most powerful ways of overcoming entrenched cultural prejudice and persuading groups to move beyond conflict into the active, energetic phase of group work. Based on Covey's work on personal development,[13] the rule states that 'you cannot make your point until you restate the point of the other person to his or her satisfaction'. This rule can be applied equally to subgroups that have taken different positions on an issue. It is a supreme test of listening skills, as Mahatma Gandhi realised: 'Most of the miseries of the world will disappear if we step into the shoes of our adversaries and understand their standpoint'.

7 Attempt role negotiation

However, there are times when both individuals and groups become 'stuck' in conflict and find it very difficult to resolve the issues. If the problems are between individuals within a group it is probably best to try to handle the problem outside the group dynamic. One of the most useful techniques for resolving conflict of this nature is role negotiation (*see* Box 8.4), which has been developed by Roger Harrison.[14] The method rests on two principles:

1   that a negotiated settlement is preferable to a situation of unresolved argument
2   that it is better (and easier) to concentrate on the adapting behaviours rather than to delve into the psychodynamic constructs that are also operating in most situations of conflict.

The method also involves commitment on the part of both individuals to engage in the process, and to understand that concessions will be required. The basic steps are shown in Box 8.4.

Box 8.4:   Role negotiation (adapted from Harrison)[14]

Each protagonist:

1   is interviewed separately
2   completes a negotiation schedule
3   meets with the facilitator to negotiate a behavioural agreement (written)
4   agrees to meet the facilitator regularly to review the agreement.

Although the negotiation method was devised to address conflict between individuals, it can be adapted for use in situations where groups disagree and fragment. It can also be used to enable so-called 'healthy' groups to gain more understanding of group dynamics. In the latter case, the process can either mirror that outlined in Box 8.4 or use the Johari window technique.[15] Using the Johari tool (*see* Chapter 10, p. 164), each group member reveals on a work-sheet the elements of their character that are 'known to self, but not known to others', in order to increase the group's insight about each member.

8 Encourage dialogue

The word 'dialogue' is usually taken to mean the type of communication or interaction that occurs between two people. However, the original roots of the word, '*dia*' and '*logos*' (Greek for 'through' and 'word', respectively) have been used by Bohm[16] to convey the concept of achieving a deep and shared understanding by any number of people. He described dialogue as a situation where conversations are quests for meaning without regard to a particular outcome. The aim is to understand the issues fully, even if this means holding on to two apparently conflicting views of the problem.

This approach requires a willingness to suspend judgement until the issues have been seen from all viewpoints. Proponents of this type of dialogue argue that when the full range of opinion has surfaced, only then are the opportunities for real and meaningful change revealed. Isaacs has outlined the purposes of dialogue as follows:[17]

- to create a 'container' (a place or situation) which enables a genuine meeting of minds
- to allow a free flow of meaning and exploration of thought, personal predisposition and collective assumptions
- to explore the experience of meaning that is embodied in a group of people.

The principles of dialogue are listed in Table 8.5.

Table 8.5:   Principles of dialogue (adapted from Isaacs)[17]

- Assumptions are made apparent
- Meaning rather than facts or ideas is valued
- Collective experience and learning are rewards in themselves
- Differences are sought and explanations attempted
- The 'container' should be large enough to accommodate the group's diversity
- Taboo subjects can be raised safely
- There is no agenda
- Direction occurs as a product of seeking meaning
- Fragmented ideas can be organised into a whole
- Complex problems are viewed in new ways
- Cross-talk is discouraged (*see* section below on 'no cross-talk' technique)
- There is a definite beginning, but no end. The 'harvest' is not hurried

9 Impose a 'no cross-talk' rule

This powerful technique (*see* Box 8.5) is taken from the conversational practices of organisations such as Alcoholics Anonymous. It firmly establishes the rule of non-judgemental sequenced contributions. Your presence at the group where 'no cross-talk' rules operate implies that you accept the powerful group norm which enables members to share their ideas without being judged or attacked.

Box 8.5:   The 'no cross-talk' rule

No cross-talk means sharing your experiences, concerns, feelings, opinions and hopes related to a particular issue without referring to or reacting to any other group member's contribution, and without evaluating what has previously been said

---

This ethos encourages the voicing of personal experiences, emotions and opinions, and is a useful mechanism for supporting individuals who have problems such as addictions. The technique can also help a group to explore a topic in more depth and from different perspectives. For instance, many facilitators use the method before a nominal group process to clarify feelings and positions related to a specific topic.

Productivity and performance

Productivity and performance in a group setting rely on many factors, ranging from the characteristics of individual members and the structural aspects of the group (status relationships and cohesiveness) to the task and environmental characteristics. These factors influence the way in which members interact with one another as they carry out their tasks. A group's effectiveness can be measured in relation to Hackman's normative model, which asks the following questions.[18]

* Does the group meet the performance standards of people who review its output?
* Has the group maintained the ability of its members to work together in the future?
* Has the group satisfied the personal needs of its individual members?

Groups do not automatically do better than individuals working alone (*see* Chapter 1, p. 18). Most research into group performance has concentrated on 'poor productivity', and has used the term 'process loss' to focus on the factors that lead to this phenomenon. Two aspects of the group process may lead to under-performance within groups, namely a lack of co-ordination and the dwindling of motivation. Loss of co-ordination is likely to occur when groups are large and need to integrate many unrelated tasks. Motivational loss (also known as 'social loafing') is the tendency for group members to exert less individual effort when working together than when working alone. Box 8.6 summarises the ways in which social loafing can be mitigated.

Box 8.6:   Ways to avoid social loafing

- Make sure that individual contributions are identifiable and unique
- Increase the transparency of individual contributions and the ease of measurement of their effect on the group performance
- Increase the accountability and involvement of individuals in the task goals
- Modify the task and increase its attractiveness and rewards

---

However, the good news is that groups can also improve their performance, and that people will often work harder when they are engaged within a group process. Interestingly, it is thought that this trend, termed 'social compensation', occurs most often when the individuals in a group think that their co-workers will not contribute adequately to what is perceived at an individual level to be an important task. This finding has an important bearing on how group productivity and member satisfaction can potentially be enhanced.

It has been demonstrated that groups set lower standards for members than individuals set for themselves, and that this goal-setting exercise significantly influences the five facets of group process (effort, planning, maintenance of internal relationships, co-operation and morale).[19] Given that the research on groups indicates that productivity is generally impeded by the normative process, it seems odd that there has been such an emphasis on teams in all aspects of organisations recently.[20,21] However, it seems that the findings of 'small group' research (usually conducted in laboratory-type settings) cannot be automatically assumed to apply to teams.[22] Teams should be regarded as a special variety of a small group – they have well-defined norms, roles and status systems.[23] As Levine points out, 'team members' self-definitions are influenced by their team affiliation'.[24] Perhaps the most important determinant of the productivity benefits within teams is the fact that team members' rewards are often associated with their team's achievement, and that successful teams are recognised within organisations as platforms enabling individuals to achieve leadership positions.

It follows therefore that, apart from the characteristics listed above which differentiate teams from groups, the mechanisms that have been developed to enhance productivity within this special type of small group involve two main techniques. First, members should participate in goal setting, and second and more recently, the importance of contributing to task design has been recognised. Providing opportunities for teams to suggest alternative ways of accomplishing tasks and encouraging processes to be entirely redesigned has allowed significant advances to be made in many organisations.[25]

From these ideas stem the myriad of techniques for improving team performance. Team development involves defining problems, negotiating agreements and achieving role clarity. Quality circles are self-managed teams who monitor the standard of their work. They require regular meetings to agree and resolve issues which impair production activities, and the concept of the self-managing or autonomous work group needs individuals to integrate interdependent tasks in order to achieve agreed outcomes. Although these developments have perhaps been most evident perhaps within industry and commerce, their parallels are seen in education, where self-directed and problem-based learning initiatives are taken up and increasingly integrated with on-line distance-learning techniques.

References

1   Wilke HAM and Meertens R (1994) *Group Performance*. Routledge, London.

2   Wit AP and Wilke HAM (1997) Interacting in task groups. In: ODW Hargie (ed) *The Handbook of Communication Skills*. Routledge, London.

3   Jackson JM and Williams KD (1985) Social loafing on difficult tasks. *J Person Psychol*. **49**: 937–42.

4   Schein E (1988) *Process Consultation* (2e). Addison-Wesley, Reading, MA.

5   Reddy BW (1994) *Intervention Skills: Process Consultation for Small Groups*. Pfeiffer & Company, San Diego, CA.

6   Harvey JB (1996) *The Abilene Paradox and Other Meditations on Management*. Jossey-Bass Publishers, San Francisco, CA.

7   Daniels WR (1987) *Group Power II: A Manager's Guide to Conducting Regular Meetings*. American Consulting and Training, Mill Valley, CA.

8   Justice T and Jamieson DW (1999) *The Facilitator's Fieldbook*. American Management Association Communications, AMA Publications, New York.

9   McGartland G (1994) *Thunderbolt Thinking*. Bernard-Davis, Austin, TX.

10 Idon Software Ltd (1996) *Idon Magnetic Hexagons*. Idon Software Ltd, Pitlochry.

11 Benne K and Sheats P (1948) The functional roles of group members. *J Soc Issues*. **4**: 42–7.

12 Crumb F (1987) *The Magic of Conflict*. Simon and Schuster, New York.

13 Covey SR, Merrill AR and Merril RR (1994) *First Things First*. Simon and Schuster, New York.

14 Harrison R (1983) When power conflicts trigger team spirit. In: WL French, CH Bell and RA Zawacki (eds) *Organization Development: Theory, Practice, Research*. Zawacki Business Publications Inc., Plano, TX.

15 Luft J (1961) The Johari window. *Hum Relations Training News*. **5**: 6–7.

16 Bohm D (1990) *On Dialogue*. David Bohm Seminars, Ojai, CA.

17 Isaacs WN (1993) Taking flight: dialogue, collective thinking, and organisational learning. *Organis Dynamics*. **2** (Autumn).

18 Hackman JR and Oldham GR (1980) *Work Redesign*. Prentice Hall Business Publishing, Englewood Cliffs, NJ.

19 O'Leary-Kelly AM, Martocchio JJ and Frink DD (1994) A review of the influence of group goals on group performance. *Acad Manag J*. **37**: 1285–301.

20 West M (1994) *Effective Teamwork*. British Psychological Society, Leicester.

21 Dyer WG (1994) *Team Building*. Addison-Wesley, Reading, MA.

22 Guzzo RA and Shea GP (1992) Group performance and interrelations in organisations. In: MD Dunnete and LM Hough (eds) *Handbook of Industrial and Organisational Psychology*. Consulting Psychologists Press, Palo Alto, CA.

23 Guzzo RA and Salas E (1995) *Team Effectiveness and Decision-Making in Organizations*. Jossey-Bass, San Francisco, CA.

24 Levine JM and Moreland RL (1998) Small groups. In: *The Handbook of Social Psychology*. McGraw-Hill, Boston, MA.

25 Hammer M and Champy J (1993) *Re-engineering the Corporation: a Manifesto For Business Revolution*. Nicholas Brearley Publishing, London.

9

Evaluating the group process

> *People ask you for criticism, but they only want praise.*
> Somerset Maugham, *Of Human Bondage*

What is evaluation and what is it for?

The term 'evaluation' means different things to different people, and this chapter is not intended to be prescriptive for all groups in all circumstances. Box 9.1 gives some general aims of an evaluation of group process. We recognise that the time and resources provided for evaluation are sometimes inadequate to cover all of these aims fully, and judgements will sometimes need to be made about priority areas.

Box 9.1: Aims of an evaluation of group process

- To enable group members to understand the process of interaction that occurred in the session
- To enable individual members to become aware of their own strengths, weaknesses, inhibitions and styles of thinking and working
- To consider possible alternative approaches to particular aspects of the session
- To promote a culture of mutual support
- To appreciate that 'normative' pressures can stifle understanding and innovation, and to ensure that effective decision-making techniques are employed within the group process
- To assist the group in moving towards a more advanced stage of development (e.g. to enable the group to reflect on a 'storming' episode and establish clearer rules of engagement)

Evaluation can be a two-edged sword. Although cynics might say that evaluation is designed to confirm predetermined judgements, there are instances where evaluation, particularly when carried out by a third party and where participants are free to comment, will lay bare many previously unidentified weaknesses and problems. Before embarking on an evaluation of group process, as in any other exercise, we therefore need to be clear about the purpose and design our tools accordingly. As Breakwell has summarised, there are three fundamental purposes to evaluation:[1]

1   to validate – to gain approval and acceptance of the status quo. This is an affirming process and gains justification both for the activity and for continuing
2   to improve – to recognise that although current practice is acceptable, it is important to identify the weak areas that can be changed
3   to condemn – to describe and highlight poor practice or processes and to prove that what exists is inadequate.

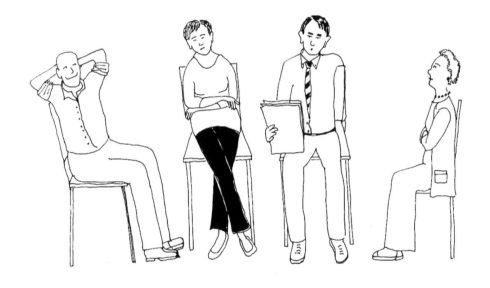

▼
Evaluating the group process.

What does evaluation of small groups encompass?

People external to a group tend to evaluate its effectiveness in terms of the group's visible products. For example, they might ask the following questions.

*   Have the students learned the material on the syllabus to the standard expected in the examination?
*   Has the committee actioned the items on the agenda?

- Has the research strategy group produced a research strategy?
- Has the fundraising group raised any funds?
- Has the teambuilding day 'built the team'?
- Did the series of focus groups of parents of children with terminal illness increase our understanding of how such parents feel, and did they inform the design of services?

These task- or product-oriented questions are, of course, highly relevant, and no one could argue that a group has been 'successful' if it has consistently failed either to deliver on its main objectives or to justify altering them! However, it is clear that many different aspects of small group work can potentially be evaluated, and there will be times when more than one aspect requires examination. For example, one could choose to evaluate any of the following:

- *process* – this can range from evaluating how a small part of the group process was conducted to the overall assessment of the process, from formation to closing.
- *people* – how did members perform, either as individuals or within their roles as participants?
- *resources* – were the allocated space, equipment, time and information adequate?
- *organisation* – did the group structure, organisational context, communication channels and organisational culture help or hinder task achievement?
- *objectives* – were the goals appropriate and did the group have a role in setting, agreeing and adapting the goals?

This chapter is mainly concerned with evaluating the group process (*see* Box 9.1). Questions you may seek to ask include the following.

- How well have the individuals engaged with one another and with the task?
- Are the roles adopted by the members appropriate?
- Has conflict been resolved or simply repressed?
- Has the final decision been reached by consensus, negotiation or domination of weaker members?
- Is the group able consistently to solve problems and/or create solutions?
- Has the group moved from hierarchical to autonomous mode (*see* Chapter 4, p. 54)?

An evaluation of the group process can include both 'formative' techniques (i.e. those which occur as you go along and which are designed specifically to improve in an additive fashion) and 'summative' techniques (i.e. those which occur in protected time at the end of a session or series, and which result in an end-point determination of success or failure).

With any evaluation method, you need to make the rules very clear at the outset, and ensure that everyone is agreed on how to apply them (*see* Chapter 5, p. 102).

Formative ('during-the-session') evaluation methods

Individual feedback

The techniques for giving personal feedback to individual group members are discussed in Chapter 4 (*see* p. 68).

The 'time-out' technique

Formative evaluation requires a means of commenting on process that is distinct from routine input on content. In other words, it is necessary to find a way for members to flag up 'I'm about to comment not on *what* we're discussing, but on *how* we're going about our discussion'. The medical faculty at McMaster University in Canada, which pioneered small group work in the postgraduate education of doctors, borrowed the expression 'time out' from baseball (*see* Table 4.3 in Chapter 4, p. 58) to describe this process.[2] It works like this. At any point during the group discussion, any group member or the facilitator may use an agreed hand signal (e.g. making a 'T' sign) and say 'time out'. He or she then makes a comment on an aspect of the group process, to which other members may respond. When the discussion on process is complete (or has been deferred by agreement), one person (perhaps the same individual who called the time out) makes another hand signal and says 'time in' to restart the discussion on content.

For example, the following dialogue is taken from a learning set of nurses addressing absenteeism in junior staff. A formative evaluation dialogue might run as follows.

Facilitator:	Has anyone else got an example of a student who repeatedly fails to turn up?
Graham:	We've got one on our ward at the moment. She arrives up to an hour late, has a fag in the toilet, and then yawns continually while on duty.
Jean:	I agree with what you're saying about that student, Graham, but you and I both know she's got personal difficulties.

Graham:	Yes, how is Lucy's father?
Jean:	He's having chemotherapy and the outlook isn't too good. She has to get up three times at night to give him his medication, and her mum doesn't help at all.
Sharon:	Oh yes, you were telling us about that girl last night. It's awful, isn't it? I was upset when my dog died of cancer – and that was only an animal.
Facilitator:	*Time out*. We were discussing absenteeism, and we were trying to think of ways to reduce that in our student nurses. Now we've heard about one young woman's personal difficulties and got side-tracked into the awfulness of people dying of cancer. How do you all feel about where the discussion is going?
Sanjay:	I think we were going a bit off track, but it does show that we need to take people's personal circumstances into account. We could use the case of Lucy to learn some general lessons about the problems some students have at home, and try and devise ways of accommodating them where appropriate.
Sally:	Yes, why don't we try to see what might help with Lucy's absenteeism problem, and then see if anything we come up with is generalisable?
Facilitator:	Okay. Let's try that. *Time in*.
Sharon:	Graham, have you sat down with Lucy and talked about her difficulties? Etc.

In our own experience, the time-out method of evaluation works well in a cohesive group whose members understand the rules, but it may cause anxiety or resentment among members who are new to group work and/or unable to conceptualise the difference between process and content (i.e. those whose 'waterline' is high; *see* Figure 8.1 in Chapter 8, p. 132).

Video playback

This is another useful 'formative' technique. The group session is videotaped and played back in sections for members to analyse 'what was going on' at different stages. Apart from technical equipment and competence, this technique does not require any special training and is probably underused. The immediacy and authenticity of the video feedback can be a powerful stimulus to learning and change.

Summative ('after-the-session') techniques

Most experienced facilitators like to allocate protected time at the end of a session in order to assess 'how it went'. It is vitally important to allocate adequate time. Jacques lists a number of methods that can be used to contribute to an after-the-session evaluation.[3] These include the following:

- *observation* – either by a single observer or using the 'fishbowl' technique in which an inner circle of participants is evaluated by an outer circle of observers
- *diaries* – in which group members record their impressions of the group process and the content covered
- *reporting back* – in which time is allocated at the beginning of a meeting for one or two members to summarise and comment on the previous session
- *checklists* – with a structured set of questions that address chosen aspects of process and content – either 'taken off the peg' (for example, *see* p. 153), or constructed *de novo* by the group
- *interviews* – in which an external assessor administers a semi-structured questionnaire to each participant
- *pass-round questionnaire* – in which each member lists (a) the things they found most valuable (and why), (b) the things they found least valuable and (c) ideas for improvements. Each list is passed successively round the group for other members to add their comments before the lists are collected together.

Process review and evaluation

Process reviews (*see* Chapter 8, p. 130) should be conducted at regular intervals during group work. When undertaken at the forming stage they can help to guide the style and methods of facilitation. A useful and very rapid technique (although potentially destructive if applied insensitively) is to divide a flipchart into two columns and mark them as 'positive' and 'negative'. The group then contributes comments or uses 'Post-It' notes to display things that have gone well or badly. A similar approach is to ask the group what they would like 'more of' and 'less of'. This may allow a gentler type of feedback. The facilitator should use this focus on the process in many creative ways. For instance, it is likely that the responsibility for at least part of any dissatisfaction or problems that surface will rest with the members of the group, and this opportunity to make the issues more transparent may well yield solutions as well.

More detailed process reviews can also be conducted, and the list of questions suggested in Box 9.2 can often help to uncover some issues if people lack experience in analysing group processes.

Box 9.2:   Process review list

Please answer yes or no to the following questions   *Yes No*

Group members are working well together   ❑   ❑
Group members are allowing everyone to participate   ❑   ❑
There is a good balance between content and process in this group   ❑   ❑
There is a good decision-making process in place in this group   ❑   ❑
There are no personality conflicts in this group   ❑   ❑
The ground rules are respected by all the members of this group   ❑   ❑
There are effective ways of recording our discussions and agreements ❑   ❑
There is a good sense of purpose and progress within the group   ❑   ❑
There are important but unresolved issues that need attention   ❑   ❑

One important but little used technique for process evaluation is analysis of the seating plan (*see* p. 42) and the sociogram (i.e. a symbolic map of who is interacting with whom) (*see* Figure 9.1 and Box 9.3).

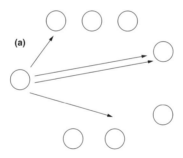

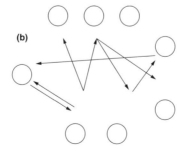

Figure 9.1:   Sociogram for a training group (a) at the outset of a session and (b) one hour into the session.

Problems with evaluation

Evaluation should be a positive experience that enables both the individual and the group to move forward. Occasionally, however, it is experienced as a negative process, and if this is the case it is probably due to one of the following four reasons.

Evaluation is viewed as an external process

As we explained in Chapter 2 (*see* p. 24), the culture in which a group operates is a crucial determinant of the group dynamics. Members who join a group may bring with them expectations and preconceptions about the nature and purpose of evaluation, which may be based on what goes on at their home institution (or even on what went on at school many years ago!). If these members are allowed to set the culture of evaluation, the group will suffer.

The 'external' approach considers that evaluation:

- is the job of an outside agent
- is separate from both the dynamics and the 'real' tasks of the group
- should be complex, technical and formal
- aims to identify poor performers with a view to penalising them
- is summative (i.e. it occurs as a final event after the work is complete)
- must be quantitative – only statistics count.

A more flexible, formative and (usually) productive approach considers that evaluation:

- is everyone's job and requires collaboration and trust
- is 'real work' and part of the task, not a 'bolt-on extra'
- should be simple, accessible and fairly informal
- aims to inform the group process, guide internal development and identify methods of achieving objectives more effectively
- is formative (i.e. it occurs as an ongoing process throughout the life of the group)
- may be qualitative (i.e. it seeks a deeper understanding of why something happens, rather than merely measuring the extent of the problem).

Individualistic behaviour dominates the group evaluation

Commercial, educational and professional groups can all become victims of the rising tide of consumerism and accountability in our society. Delegates on courses, students, and clients of the service sector are all increasingly demanding 'value for money' (*see* the section on 'personal baggage' in Chapter 2,

p. 23). Rights are often given more prominence than responsibilities, and people who have made a considerable personal or financial sacrifice in order to attend a group may unconsciously be more concerned about what they expect to get out of the group than about what they can put into it. This is especially true if the group members have a passive view of learning and feel that it is the facilitator's role to impart facts. In such situations, the evaluation session can quickly degenerate into a complaints session directed predominantly at the facilitator.

Too much evaluation is attempted

Excessive evaluation can be tedious and artificial, and can inhibit the development of the group. This may be particularly the case when interaction is flagging and the group seems to be 'stuck'. In such situations, it may be more appropriate to allow communication to flow so that interaction picks up naturally, rather than to impose a 'navel-gazing' session.

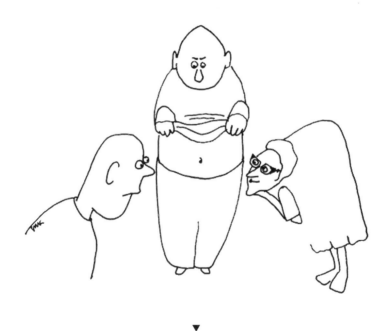

▼
A navel-gazing session.

Evaluation divides the group

An evaluation that rewards some members of the group while penalising others will unwittingly divide the group, especially if factions are already forming. Even when one group member has led the session, evaluation should always address the group's performance as well as that of the designated leader. If a session is perceived to have gone badly, the group must take some responsibility and reflect on how the lead member might have been supported better.

One sure way to kill group interaction is to tell students or trainees that they will be assessed individually on the content of their contributions. In an early series of experiments on the group process, Deutsch gave groups different information on how they would be assessed. Participants who believed that they were being assessed by the whole group's performance showed more interaction, greater co-ordination of effort, more attentiveness to fellow members, and more productivity per unit time compared to participants who thought that they were being assessed individually. They also evaluated the group and its products more favourably.[4]

For all of the above reasons, it is important to address the issue of evaluation in the first group session, and to set ground rules for what is to be evaluated, why and how.

Box 9.3:   Checklist for evaluating a group session

The questions below have been adapted from a number of previously published sources[5–10] as well as previously unpublished checklists of our own.

Objectives and setting
1   Were objectives clear, appropriate, understood by all members and agreed? (*See* p. 149)
2   Was the physical setting appropriate? Who sat where? (*See* Figure 9.1, p. 153)
3   Was enough time allocated, and was good use made of the time available? (*See* p. 149)
4   Was the atmosphere open, trusting and supportive? (*See* p. 97)
5   Were members adequately prepared? (*See* p. 115)

Participation
6   Who did the talking, and to whom was it directed? (*See* Figure 9.1, p. 153)
7   Did everyone have their say, and was everyone listened to? (*See* p. 152)
8   Was conflict suppressed or successfully resolved (and if so, how)? (*See* p. 129)
9   Did individual aims interfere with the group? (*See* p. 144)

Roles and rules
10   What role did each member play? (*See* p. 137)
11   Were roles fixed or changing, negotiable or imposed? (*See* pp. 124–5)
12   What was the pattern of power and influence? (*See* pp. 124–5)
13   What rules for individual behaviour were adopted? (*See* p. 97)

continued opposite

Task
14 Were members committed to the task? (*See* p. 149)
15 Were creative ideas suggested and taken up? (*See* p. 73)
16 Were individual members' skills identified and used appropriately? (*See* p. 73)
17 Did the group achieve its task objectives? (*See* p. 149)

Facilitation
18 What role did the facilitator play? (*See* Chapter 4, p. 49)
19 What proportion of time did the facilitator talk for? (*See* p. 153)
20 What techniques did he or she use to involve (and, if necessary, control) group members? (*See* p. 49)

References

1 Breakwell G and Millward L (1995) *Basic Evaluation Methods: Analysing Perform-ance, Procedure and Practice*. British Psychologist Society, Leicester.

2 Donald A (1994) *Evidence-Based Medicine: a Report From McMaster University Medical School and Teaching Hospitals: Becoming Better, Faster, Happier Docs*. Anglia and Oxford Regional Health Authority, Oxford.

3 Jacques D (1991) *Learning in Groups* (2e). Kogan Page, London.

4 Deutsch M (1949) Experimental study of effects of co-operation and competition on group process. *Human Relations*.

5 Jacques D (1991) *ibid*, pp. 177–80.

6 University Teaching Methods Unit (1978) *Improving Teaching in Higher Education*. University Teaching Methods Unit, London.

7 Tiberius R (1999) *Small Group Teaching – a Troubleshooting Guide*. Kogan Page, London.

8 Entwhistle N, Thompson S and Tait H (1992) *Guidelines for Promoting Effective Learning in Higher Education*. Centre for Research on Learning and Instruction, Edinburgh.

9 Reynolds M (1994) *Group Work in Education and Training*. Kogan Page, London.

10 Derived from Schein EH (1988) *Process Consultation: its role in organization development. Vol 1* (2e). Addison-Wesley, New York.

10

When groups go wrong

Stop saying nothing in such an aggressive voice.
Mel Calman, *A Little Light Worrying*

As other chapters in this book indicate, group work can be both satisfying and productive. However, when things go wrong, the group experience can be frustrating, demotivating and even depressing. This chapter describes the common symptoms of the dysfunctional group, considers some causes, and explores some potential methods for troubleshooting.

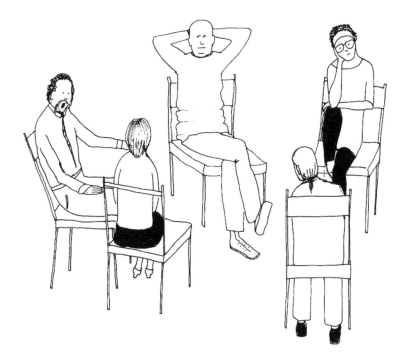

▼
When groups go wrong.

How do you know that your group is dysfunctional?

Box 10.1 gives some examples of groups going wrong. Sometimes the dysfunctional nature of the interaction is only evident with hindsight, or members only become aware of it when someone calls attention to process issues (*see* p. 129).

Box 10.1:   Examples of groups 'going wrong'

An academic lecturer is asked to come and lead a two-hour session with 15 undergraduate students from a different department. The students all know each other but the lecturer knows no one. The lecturer divides the group into triads and asks them to think about three written questions. It soon becomes clear that they are not even attempting the set task. Some of them are chatting about last night's television and others are looking vacant.

Five general practitioners and one community nurse, together with three representatives of advocacy and self-help organisations, have volunteered to produce a draft local strategy for supporting mentally ill patients in the community. They have met four times, but almost everyone experiences the meetings as unproductive and disheartening. Several members have produced written suggestions, and one of the GPs has volunteered to 'pull it all together'. However, although all of the suggestions are good ones, they don't fit together and some even conflict with one another. There is a general feeling of irritation and confusion, and much whispering between factions outside the group.

A health authority subcommittee with six members is given a brief to oversee an audit of referrals to a specialist cancer unit for a forthcoming public report. The data are already available, and the task seems straightforward. However, at the first three meetings attendance is very poor, with no more than three people turning up each time. On each occasion, different members fail to turn up, which creates difficulties when work to date is reviewed and new tasks are allocated. The chairman, who is relatively junior in the organisation, suspects that several senior members of the group are avoiding each other following a previous high-profile confrontation on another project. Two people in particular are said to have 'difficult personalities' and are not 'team players'.

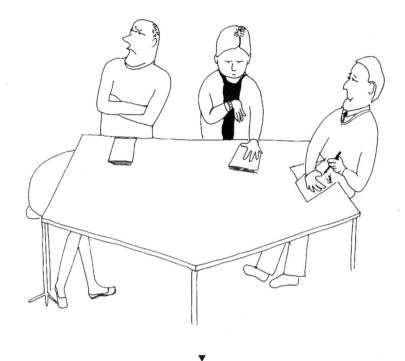

▼

How do you know that your group is dysfunctional?

If a group or team is not working, the following symptoms may be particularly prevalent:

1   *frustration* – individuals find it difficult to meet their own needs and fulfil their aspirations. For example, they may feel that they are being punished for mistakes, rather than mistakes being used as opportunities for the team to learn. High levels of negative emotion are common in this situation

2   *unhealthy competition* – backbiting, dirty tricks and internal politics become prominent features, and the group repeatedly misses opportunities because of such behaviour

3   *body language* – frustrated individuals lack motivation and commitment. This often shows on their faces and in the rush to clock off!

4   *dishonesty, secretiveness and mistrust* – individuals revert to protecting their own territory, and interpersonal relationships within and beyond the group are characterised by antipathy, resentment, locked drawers and locked doors

5   *poor use of meetings* – these are used as an opportunity to lay down rules rather than utilising the collective skills of the group to work on a common problem or opportunity

6   *isolated absent leader* – the leader becomes isolated from the group and no longer represents or subscribes to the group's views

7   *lack of group or personal development* – for a group or team to be effective, it and the individuals within it need to be constantly developing. Development may be hindered by the following:
- perceived or real time pressures
- conflict between the team and organisational culture
- development being perceived as the job of the personnel or training function
- the team leader lacking the skills or willingness to make it happen
- fear of the consequences of team development.

Why is the group performing poorly?

The reasons for poor group work can be broadly divided into seven categories, which are considered in turn below:

1   members behave inappropriately
2   members have hidden agendas
3   one or more members are dysfunctional
4   the group becomes too comfortable and uncritical (groupthink)
5   the group has not developed properly
6   the group has been established inappropriately
7   the group has been poorly facilitated.

Members behave inappropriately

In Chapter 4 (*see* pp. 58–68), we gave examples of difficult roles that group members may take on, including the digressor, the know-all and the joker. However, once a group starts to become dysfunctional, unhelpful behaviour can be (and often is) exhibited by all of the group members and even by the facilitator! Box 10.2 lists some behaviours which can inhibit and block the work of groups. It is adapted from a list produced by John Hunt, with additional input from our own experience.

Box 10.2:   Dysfunctional group behaviours (adapted from Hunt)[1]

Changing the topic: Changing the focus from one topic to another, or from one person to another.

Digressing: Failing to stick to the issue being discussed, similar to 'changing the topic', but one usually finds that it is the member's favourite subject that is raised repeatedly.

continued opposite

Dominating: One group member dominates all of the group meetings and does not allow others to make an equal contribution. This behaviour can include shutting others out or talking over them. It also includes interrupting behaviour. At its extreme this behaviour becomes 'Fight' (described below).

Entertaining: One member spends most of their time joking and making no attempt to contribute any sensible material to the discussion. This may be because that group member has a poor understanding of the topic, is embarrassed, or finds it difficult to argue his or her case.

Expertise: Blocking contrary arguments by 'dropping' data about one's own expertise (e.g. 'When I was in Paris, the Minister was saying to me...'). It may include using legal or scientific jargon to dazzle.

Fight: Win–lose conflicts that are difficult to resolve.

Flight: Running away, which sometimes involves actually leaving the group. More frequently it is displayed as 'sulk' behaviour or withdrawal (e.g. leaving the room, pretending to sleep, sitting back from the table, or saying 'I'm not really interested in the question').

Holding back: A group member implies that he or she knows the answer to a group problem, but is not going to tell it to the group.

Lying: Deliberate distortion of the facts in order to preserve a position in the group.

Making noise: Speaking to be heard rather than to contribute (often very fuzzy and undisciplined). This behaviour is commonly displayed in training groups.

Pairing: Breaking into subgroups rather than solving the conflict as a group coalition.

Put-downs: Verbal or physical aggression towards others, which can considerably alter the dynamics of the group. Putting oneself down may generate sympathy and diffuse the opposition (the 'poor me' game).

Seeking attention: Asking questions to which one already knows the answer. This is usually done to ensure that the member has as much 'airtime' as possible and can demonstrate how clever they are.

Suppressing emotions: Rather than letting the emotional blockages out, a group member demands logic and rationality (e.g. 'Let's not get emotional' or 'Please let's act like adults'). This is unfortunate, as blockage is often emotional and should generally be expressed.

If you recognise any of these behaviours in your group, it is important to raise the individual's and the group's awareness of them. In many cases, the individual will not be aware of what they are doing, and the group may need help in addressing the problem. *Feedback* – defined as information communicated

		SELF	
		Known	*Not known*
OTHERS	*Known*	Public self	Blind self
	Not known	Private self	Unknown

Figure 10.1:   Johari window model of individual performance.

to a group member about his or her performance – is one way of addressing this. If giving and receiving feedback is to be a useful developmental tool, then there must be an atmosphere of openness and trust between the group members and the facilitator, as discussed in Chapter 4 (*see* p. 68).

The *Johari window* model (*see* Figure 10.1) is used in management to conceptualise the feedback process, and to enable individuals to identify both their strengths and their development needs.

We all have aspects of our performance that could be improved, and of which no one is yet aware. Working in a group may reveal these areas of potential improvement to our fellow group members – that is, allow us to move from the bottom right-hand corner of the matrix in Figure 10.1 ('unknown') to the top right-hand corner ('blind self'). Feedback delivered in a confidential and trusting environment (*see* Chapter 4, p. 71) allows us to move safely to the left-hand side of the matrix and begin to develop action and development plans to improve our performance. Sharing what we know or suspect about our own performance (i.e. moving from the 'private self' to the 'public self' via self-disclosure to the group) may also help us to begin a process of learning and change, as shown in Figure 10.2.

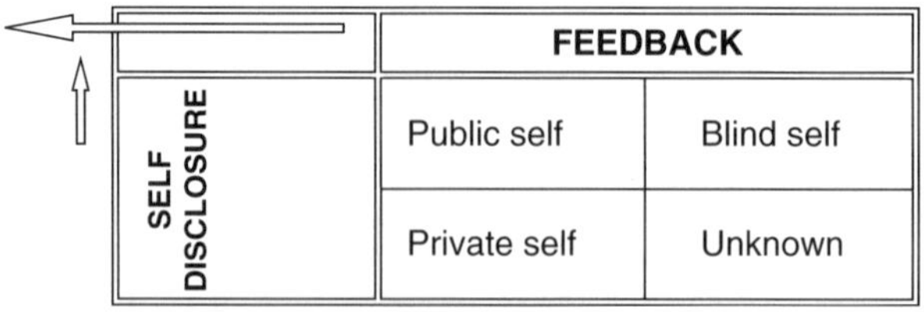

		FEEDBACK	
SELF DISCLOSURE		Public self	Blind self
		Private self	Unknown

Figure 10.2:   Johari window showing effect of feedback and self-disclosure.

Members have hidden agendas

It is common sense that if all members of a group share the same objectives the group will tend to be that much more effective. However, this state of affairs is rarely found in real life. In most groups there is some degree of conflict between individual and group objectives, and compromise is required (*see* Chapter 8, p. 137). When individuals come together in a group, there should be an agenda-setting exercise at the outset to define and agree on group objectives (*see* p. 78). Those individuals whose stated personal objectives cannot be reconciled with the group's agreed objectives have a difficult choice – either to put up with the situation or leave the group.

However, the main problem with conflicting objectives is not usually the stated ones – which can be acknowledged and negotiated – but the unstated or hidden (and perhaps unconscious) objectives ('baggage') that people bring to groups (*see* Chapter 2, p. 23). Hidden agendas can override the individual's motivation to contribute to the group process – and they frequently cause major disruption within the group. These agendas can cover a range of territory, including the following:

- protecting one's own (undeclared) interests
- impressing others (motives may include enhancing prospects for promotion, overcoming personal inadequacy, or sexual desire)
- trying to put down an opponent or colleague (perhaps with similar motives)
- building a particular alliance
- covering up errors
- avoiding taking on extra work.

If you suspect that hidden agendas are influencing your group, it is essential to try to bring them out into the open. It is also vital that all members are clear about the group's objectives and the benefits that they will bring. The facilitator may need to confront individuals who appear to be more committed to conflicting objectives.

One or more members are dysfunctional

We all have good days and bad days, and some of our group experiences are better than others. We also all have a natural tendency to adopt particular roles in a group (*see* Chapter 16, p. 261). However, some individuals are, to put it mildly, not 'team players' (i.e. in general, they have the types of personality that make them difficult to get along with in a group). As we explained in Chapter 4 (*see* p. 58), personality represents by definition the aspects of personhood that are difficult or impossible to change, and it is an important aspect of the group's development to identify, utilise (and, if necessary, contain) the different personality attributes of its members. However, whereas hidden agendas (see above) may be amenable to negotiation by bringing them out into the open, a 'difficult personality' cannot, in general, be altered, and must instead be contained or ejected from the group. As Chapter 4 suggests, dysfunctional behaviour can sometimes (but not always) be managed by confronting the individual outside the group.

Groupthink

Groups sometimes become too cohesive and cosy. Groupthink (first described by IL Janis)[2] occurs when too high a price is placed on the harmony and morale of the group, so that loyalty to the group's previous policies, or to the group consensus, overrides the objectives (and indeed the conscience and common sense) of each member. Janis has identified eight symptoms of groupthink:[2]

1 *invulnerability* – the group becomes over-optimistic and may take extraordinary risks without realising the dangers, mainly because there is no discordant warning voice
2 *rationale* – the group is quick to find rationalisations to explain away evidence that does not fit their policies
3 *morality* – there is a tendency to be blind to the moral or ethical implications of a policy ('How could so many good men be wicked?')
4 *stereotypes* – victims of groupthink quickly get into the habit of stereotyping their enemies or other people, and do not notice discordant evidence
5 *pressure* – if anyone starts to voice doubts, the group exerts subtle pressures to keep them quiet; they are allowed to express doubts but not to press them
6 *self-censorship* – members of the group are careful not to discuss their feelings or their doubts outside the group, in order not to disturb the group cosiness
7 *unanimity* – once a decision has been reached, any divergent views are carefully screened out of people's minds
8 *mindguards* – victims of groupthink set themselves up as bodyguards to the decision ('He needs all the support we can give him'). The doctrine of collective responsibility is invoked in order to stifle dissent outside the group.

The result of groupthink is that the group looks at too few alternatives, is insensitive to the risks in its favourite strategy, finds it difficult to rethink a strategy that is failing, and becomes very selective about the types of facts it sees and asks for. Two well-publicised examples (*see* Boxes 10.3 and 10.4) illustrate these processes. However, it would be wrong to think of 'groupthink' as something that occurs only rarely and which produces spectacular catastrophies such as the examples in Boxes 10.3 and 10.4. The same fundamental process frequently underlies the dozens of inept and indefensible decisions that occur daily in the boardroom, the staff-room, the committee room and on the ward round.

Janis suggested that the antecedents to the groupthink syndrome are high group cohesion, directive autocratic leadership styles and a provocative situational context (e.g. an external threat).[3] All of these influences encourage the process of 'jumping to a conclusion' and then instil a closed-mindedness to any other views and an inability to consider alternative options. However, Janis's analysis has received mixed empirical support.[4]

Box 10.3:   The Bay of Pigs disaster[2]

In 1961, President John F Kennedy and a group of his closest advisers made the decision to support a small group of Cuban exiles in invading the Cuban coast. Despite the full support of the American Air Force, everything went wrong, and within a few days all of the invaders had been killed or captured. Kennedy considered making a bigger strike on Cuba and, in response, President Kruschev of the USSR launched a fleet of cargo ships containing nuclear weapons, bringing the world closer to nuclear war than it has ever been before or since.

John F Kennedy subsequently went on record as saying 'How could we have been so stupid?'. The answer, as Janis showed by a detailed analysis of the official papers, was groupthink. Kennedy and his cronies – described as one of the finest collections of intellectual and political talent in the world at the time – had become too cosy in their thinking and had abandoned their individual critical faculties.

Box 10.4:   The Challenger disaster[5]

On 28 January 1986, 15 million people world-wide tuned their television sets to watch the launch of the latest US space rocket. This was to be a particularly memorable flight, as the US government had planned (by way of a publicity exercise) to put the first 'ordinary citizen' in space. Schoolteacher Christa McAuliffe, winner of a huge national competition, watched by her husband and two small children, entered the shuttle along with six fully trained astronauts. To the outside world all appeared to be going well, and the countdown began. The rocket launched, to massive cheers, but after just six seconds it exploded dramatically, killing all of its occupants and stultifying the USA's space programme for the next 12 years.

continued overleaf

Again, groupthink was almost certainly to blame for this needless and staggeringly expensive loss of life. It subsequently emerged that the engineers had spotted the seals on the fuel containers failing at low launch temperatures, and tried to communicate this fact to senior colleagues, but no one had listened to them. A further series of ill-advised decisions led to the launch of a craft that was known to be unsafe in weather conditions which, very predictably, exacerbated the risk.

The group has not developed properly

In Chapter 1 (*see* p. 11) we introduced the stages of group development (forming, storming, norming and performing), and we discussed these stages in more detail in Chapters 6, 7 and 8. For the group to be effective, it is usually necessary to go through all of these stages. The development process can be emotionally draining and sometimes even painful for the members. Understandably, some groups resist it.

Most commonly, a group gets stuck at the forming or storming stage and fails to move on to the norming or performing stages. Such groups are unproductive, conflict-ridden, time-consuming and to be avoided. Group development may become arrested for any of the following reasons:

- failure to clarify or state the group's goals and secure agreement on the task
- failure to signal which individuals are members
- failure to choose suitable team tasks (e.g. attempting to address tasks that individuals are better working on alone) (*see* p. 16)
- avoiding team-building – concentrating solely on achieving the task rather than addressing how the group is performing
- meeting too infrequently
- making group meetings last too long
- failure to share materials, papers and experiences
- preferring social activities to work activities
- playing political games.

Lack of group development is more likely if members behave inappropriately, have hidden agendas or are dysfunctional but, as the list above shows, it can also occur in potentially effective groups when the context, task or external factors are wrong. These issues are discussed in more detail in Chapter 2 (*see* p. 18), Chapter 16 (*see* p. 267) and below.

The group has been established inappropriately

Sometimes, rather depressingly, a group or team discovers that it cannot do the job it has been set up to do. The members are not dysfunctional, nor are they unmotivated, but there is a general feeling that there is something inappropriate about them having come together at all. Problems may include any of the following.

Poor recruitment and selection

'Setting up a group/team/task force' is a common (and very reasonable) response to a complex problem in an organisation. Yet, despite the fact that organisations often possess a wealth of experience in the recruitment and selection of *individuals* for particular posts, they frequently come up with the wrong mix of people for a team activity. Those who are charged with setting up a team should think carefully both about the skill mix required and about the personalities of potential members (*see* p. 261). A group composed entirely of chairpeople, or of experts in one aspect of a multifaceted problem, may make remarkably slow progress!

Confused organisational structure

If a team is expected to work within an organisation, it will almost certainly be expected to follow the rules and cultural codes of that organisation (*see* pp. 24–7). For example, strongly hierarchical organisations work best when they are required to perform repetitive tasks in which they are well versed, and are working to meet rigid and regular deadlines. However, when the work being undertaken requires a high element of initiative or creativity, rigid role definition, hierarchy and an 'accountability' culture impede the process of free thought, and decision making is less effective. A hierarchical organisation that sets up a group charged with creative decision making may find that the new organism begins to break organisational rules and challenge deeply held beliefs and practices. In this situation, the group cannot produce the solution to the organisation's problems but, even so, the process may help to expose key structural faults.

Poor training

One of the essential features of an effective team is the skill and knowledge of its members – attributes that are (hopefully) continually being updated and reviewed. Group work may identify the need for individual training and development, but it will not fulfil the organisation's need to provide training for staff. It is vital to the work of the group that staff feel comfortable about identifying their learning needs and seeking further training. If a group that is set up to address a particular problem flounders because its members are inadequately trained, this could be an opportunity for the organisation to review training policy and practice.

Low motivation

The way that people feel about the organisation profoundly affects the amount of effort they are prepared to put into their working lives. Setting up a 'team-building' group when the individuals concerned have a poor view of the organisation is unlikely to improve either motivation or performance. A key aspect of motivation is the match between the aims of the organisation and those of the individual, and if there is a serious mismatch, group work should probably be avoided until this has been resolved.

Unclear aims

Teams exist to undertake tasks, and they need a clear view of where they are expected to go and why. Highly developed teams without an aim will degenerate into mere groups of people.

Unfair rewards

A team that works hard to complete its task may reasonably expect a reward from the organisation, and an individual who 'does their bit' may expect to be rewarded individually. Effective teamwork depends on a reward system that offers adequate incentives to the members to make a contribution. Rewards may not necessarily be financial or material – the fact that one's contribution 'goes on record' may be enough. Totally equitable reward systems are difficult to find, but at the very least the system must recognise variety of input and output and be felt to be fair. For example, if the team's task is to produce a report which will bear only the chairperson's name, and for which he or she stands to gain 90% of the credit, there may well be a shortage of volunteers for the actual work.

The group has been poorly facilitated

Facilitation and its problems are discussed in detail in Chapter 4 (*see* pp. 56–7). All too commonly a poor facilitator will scapegoat individual members or blame the group as a whole for a session that has gone badly. In our experience, the only way to deal with a facilitator who repeatedly derails the group with poor facilitation techniques is for a member of the group to confront him or her and take over the facilitation role. This tactic should certainly be considered if one of the other group members is sufficiently competent and has a mandate from the remainder of the group.

Conclusion: some tips for improving group performance

Most of this book is about improving group performance, and you will probably have gathered that there is no quick fix! Listed below are a number of simple strategies, which are derived from the more theoretical background covered elsewhere in this book. We hope that they will provide a helpful basis for improving the functioning of even the most uninspiring of groups.

- Ensure that the atmosphere is informal, comfortable and relaxed. There should be no obvious tensions and no signs of boredom.
- There should be plenty of discussion in which virtually everyone participates, and which is directed towards clarifying and achieving the objectives.
- The tasks or objectives of the group should be well understood and accepted by all of the members.
- The members should listen to each other and every idea should be given a hearing. People should not be afraid of appearing foolish, as all of the group members are supportive of the potential contributions of others.
- There should be room for disagreement. Disagreements are not suppressed or overridden by premature group action, and the group gains strength from conflict, rather than being weakened by it (*see* Chapter 8, p. 138).
- There is no tyranny by or of the minority. Individuals who disagree do not appear to try to dominate the group or express hostility, and the team is capable of assimilating new ideas.
- Most agreements should be reached by consensus. Voting is minimal.
- Criticism should be frank, frequent and relatively comfortable. There should be little evidence of personal attack – the group is able to integrate different ideologies, needs and goals.
- People should feel free to express their feelings as well as their ideas. There are few 'hidden agendas'.
- When action is taken, clear allocation of tasks and assignments is made and accepted. Members also accept responsibility for the work of the group.
- The chairman or leader of the group should not dominate it, nor on the other hand should the group defer unduly to him or her. The leadership

can shift from time to time, depending on the knowledge and resources within the group. There is little evidence of struggles for power.

• The group must develop the ability to make use of all the resources that are available internally within it and externally within the larger organisation. This will mean ensuring that all resources are known about.

• The group should be self-conscious about the processes within it. It will be prepared to stop to examine how well it is doing, or what may be interfering with its operation.

References

1   Hunt J (1992) *Managing People at Work – a Manager's Guide to Behaviour in Organizations* (3e). McGraw-Hill, London.

2   Janis IL (1972) *Victims of Groupthink.* Houghton-Mifflin, Boston, MA.

3   Janis IL (1982) *Groupthink: Psychological Studies of Policy Decisions and Fiascos* (2e). Houghton-Mifflin, Boston, MA.

4   Aldag RJ and Fuller SR (1993) Beyond fiasco: a reappraisal of the groupthink phenomenon and a new model of group decision processes. *Psychol Bull.* **113**: 533–52.

5   Esser JK and Lindoerfer JS (1989) Groupthink and the space shuttle Challenger accident: toward a quantitative case analysis. *J Behav Decision Making.* **2**: 167–77.

Part 3

Small group work in educational settings

11

Evidence for the effectiveness of small group work in higher education

> 'Men', said the little prince, 'set out on their way in express trains, but they do not know what they are looking for. Then they rush about, and get excited, and turn round and round...'
> Antoine de Saint-Exupery, *The Little Prince*

How do adults learn effectively?

The rote learning of facts has been the lot of the assessment-driven student since time immemorial. Over the past generation, educationalists have come to distinguish between the kind of learning that allows basic assimilation of facts and the deeper level of learning that allows the student to process those facts, link them with other areas of knowledge and apply them to new situations (*see* Table 11.1).[1]

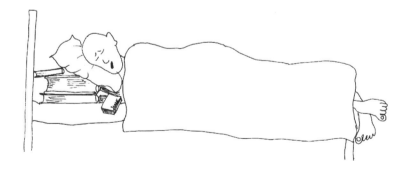

▼

Rote learning: very much in evidence in the examination system.

Rote learning, although still very much in evidence in the examination systems of schools and universities, is now recognised as an entirely different (and usually inferior) process to true learning – in which the student first identifies a lack of understanding and then converts this to understanding through active, constructive mental activity.[2] As the later part of this chapter will demonstrate, the group process promotes deep learning by encouraging higher-level activities such as reflection, analysis and evaluation.

Table 11.1:   Features of superficial and deep learning

Superficial learning	Deep learning
Comprises assimilation of facts	Comprises conversion of lack of understanding to understanding
Requires only lower-order skills (memorising, reproducing)	Requires higher-order skills (analysis, valuation, synthesis)
Essentially a passive activity	Requires active input from the student
Driven by external factors (e.g. assessment method)	Driven by reflection on own learning needs

The strong support by some adult educationalists[3] for small group methods is based on a particular theoretical model of how adults learn. The founding fathers of adult learning theory (also called the theory of experiential learning) were Kurt Lewin and John Dewey, whose work has been summarised and extended by David Kolb.[4] Both Lewin and Dewey undertook detailed observational studies in both simulated and 'real-life' learning situations. The central tenet of both their theories, and of Kolb's unifying model, is the crucial importance of personal experience in testing, validating and modifying abstract concepts.

Figure 11.1 (based on a model which most attribute to Kolb, but Kolb himself credits to Lewin) illlustrates the experiential learning cycle, which emphasises the role of active experience in shaping the concepts and generalisations that constitute understanding. Both Lewin and Kolb were convinced of the importance of *feedback* in the effective progression of the learning cycle. Lewin used an analogy borrowed from electrical engineering to illustrate how adequate, precise feedback enables the learner to assess deviation from desired goals. He demonstrated that ineffective attempts at learning were often characterised by an imbalance between observation and action. This took the form of either an excessive focus on action at the expense of information gathering, or an excessive focus on collecting and analysing data with insufficient action to test new concepts.[5]

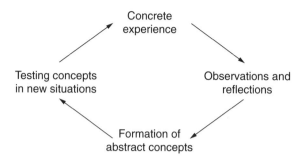

Figure 11.1: The experiential learning cycle (attributed to Lewin and Kolb).

Experiential learning theories (of which there are now several) differ fundamentally from both instructivist theories (which depict learning in terms of the accumulation of facts, e.g. storing money in a bank, and which assume that learning can be assessed by the reproduction of these facts) and behaviourist theories (which depict learning in terms of performance outputs, e.g. teaching a dog to beg for a reward, and which deny, or at least refuse to analyse, any key role of consciousness in the learning process).

First, experiential learning theories assume that facts are not fixed and immutable elements of thought, but are constantly formed and reformed through reflection and experience. Second, experiential approaches view learning as a continuous process in which every new experience builds on and integrates with the accumulated experiences that have gone before. Thus, says Kolb, no two thoughts are ever the same, since experience always intervenes.[3]

Third, and this is where the group process comes in (*see* Figure 11.2 and Box 11.1), these theories give a central importance to social discourse as a means of consolidating or changing understanding. As Freire put it, 'Knowledge emerges only through invention and reinvention, through the restless, impatient, continuing, hopeful inquiry men pursue in the world, with the world, and with each other'.[4]

A reviewer of the first draft of this book, Dr Anita Berlin, commented that the learning cycle associated with conventional theories of adult learning (*see* Figure 11.1) does not explicitly incorporate the role of the group. According to Figure 11.1, the link between reflection and the formation of new abstract concepts is a highly individual one which carries the risk of a limited frame of reference and 'navel-gazing'. Berlin suggested an additional loop in the learning cycle (*see* Figure 11.2) representing discourse with others which, if present, may increase the likelihood that reflection will lead to new and transformed meaning for the individual. This transformational potential is the 'added value' of group discussion over and above individual reflection. In addition, as discussed in Chapters 14 and 15, group work enhances motivation and provides a social and practical context for the material that is learned. The potential downside of group work for individual learning is groupthink (a shared sense of unanimity, invulnerability and moral blindness in which poor decisions are irrationally produced and fiercely defended by a group that is unconsciously avoiding conflict) (for further discussion *see* p. 231).

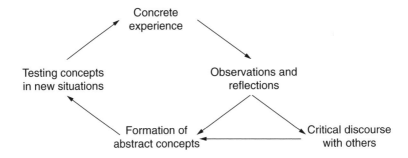

Figure 11.2:   Effect of group work on the experiential learning cycle (suggested by Anita Berlin).

Box 11.1:   Potential advantages of small group work for experiential learning

- Encourages learners to control and direct their learning
- Enables learners to identify gaps in their understanding and make connections between concepts
- Activates previously acquired understanding
- Promotes questioning and discussion
- Promotes higher-level activities conducive to deep learning (*see* Table 11.1)
- Allows application and development of ideas
- Promotes change in individual attitudes and motivation
- Improves confidence and self-esteem

Small group methods have been introduced in universities in parallel with problem-based learning (PBL) (*see* Figure 11.3). PBL is an increasingly popular educational technique which aims (among other things) to achieve deep learning.[6]

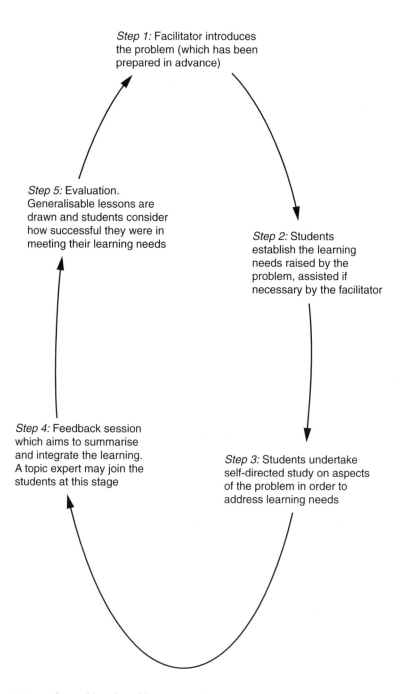

Step 1: Facilitator introduces the problem (which has been prepared in advance)

Step 5: Evaluation. Generalisable lessons are drawn and students consider how successful they were in meeting their learning needs

Step 2: Students establish the learning needs raised by the problem, assisted if necessary by the facilitator

Step 4: Feedback session which aims to summarise and integrate the learning. A topic expert may join the students at this stage

Step 3: Students undertake self-directed study on aspects of the problem in order to address learning needs

Figure 11.3:   The problem-based learning cycle.

What counts as evidence of effective education and how far can we trust that evidence?

In 1996, a new lecturer, Anna Donald, was appointed to teach clinical epidemiology to medical students in a public health department at a London medical school. Anna was a graduate of McMaster University in Canada, where small group problem-based learning had been pioneered in the 1970s.[7] Prior to Anna's appointment, the teaching of clinical epidemiology had been delivered by traditional lectures and was (according to rumour) perceived by students as a rather dull and detached part of the curriculum. Around 25% of students failed the course, and the highest mark recorded in recent years by any student had been 72%.

Within one year of Anna introducing small group teaching methods, student performance in examinations had improved dramatically, with virtually no one failing the course, and the *average* mark being around 70%. Evaluations were very positive, and anecdotal reports indicated that students could at last see the relevance of this topic to other parts of the curriculum.

Despite being justifiably proud of this success, Anna was the first person to point out that these results prove almost nothing (or at least nothing generalisable) about the effectiveness of small group work in educational settings. The introduction of the new teaching method was not intended to be a research study – Anna simply chose to teach in this way. The main reasons why we should be wary of drawing conclusions from the above story about the effectiveness of small group work *in general* are as follows.

1   Anna is an enthusiastic and skilled teacher who knows her subject well and prepares carefully for each teaching session. The improvement in marks may have been due mainly or wholly to her personal qualities, and not at all to the fact that students were placed in small groups or invited to address clinical problems rather than working through a structured syllabus.

2   Anna introduced a number of innovative techniques in addition to small group work, including learning contracts, explicit objectives for each session and self-assessment quizzes. Any one of these additional innovations could have explained the results.

3   This small 'experiment' in small group methods was not the only curriculum change at that particular medical school in 1996. In particular, the popularity of clinical epidemiology (under its new name 'evidence-based medicine') was rising rapidly and many clinical specialties were gradually incorporating the concepts of this subject into their own

topic-based teaching. Medical journals frequently contained articles about this newly fashionable subject. Thus planned changes in the taught syllabus for clinical epidemiology were occurring against a shifting baseline of acceptability and importance in the medical school as a whole (and beyond it).

4   Anna's reputation as a McMaster-trained teacher probably went before her. At least some students would have learned from their colleagues that this was a new, successful way of learning that was all the rage in North America,[7] and that the public health faculty were most interested to see whether it worked in the UK, too. A 'Hawthorne effect' was likely (i.e. students may have performed better simply because they knew they were being studied).

5   The fact that students scored better in their examinations does not *necessarily* mean that they were better able to apply the principles of clinical epidemiology in practice, or that the patients they subsequently treated would live longer or have better lives!

6   This story might not have been told at all, and would almost certainly not have been published, if the students on the new course had scored substantially lower than in previous years.

These specific caveats illustrate a number of more general problems with regard to research into adult education. These can be listed as follows.

- *Confounding.* Real-life case studies that purport to demonstrate the success of a new method of learning are often contaminated by other important (but unmeasured) factors that may have affected outcome. If such studies do not include a contemporaneous control group (i.e. if they simply describe what happened with one method, rather than comparing this with a different method used on a similar group of students), the extent of this contamination cannot be estimated.

- *External influences.* Education (especially adult education) does not occur in a social or cultural vacuum. Rather, external influences (notably changes in political and pedagogical climate, and the influence of the mass media) may profoundly affect the outcome of studies undertaken in the class-room and workplace. This potential bias is, of course, especially important if there is no control group in the study.

- *Validity of outcome measures.* The objective assessment of learning (e.g. through examinations) may not be a valid indicator of a person's under-standing of the subject or of their ability to apply what they have learned in the workplace. An improvement in examination results may reflect no more than the fact that the course has become more assessment driven.

- *Publication bias.* 'Positive' studies (i.e. those that demonstrate improved effectiveness of a new technique), even when scientifically rigorous, may be more likely to appear in reputable academic journals. There may be an equal or greater number of negative studies (which failed to demonstrate any improvement) that have not been published.

*   *Generalisability.* Every teaching situation is unique, and in 'real-life' teaching (as opposed to the controlled environment of the laboratory), outcome will be determined by a host of factors including the personality of the teacher, the background and motivation of the students, the culture of the educational institution, the nature of the wider curriculum, as well as important physical factors such as space and comfort. Although in theory these factors can be 'controlled for', in reality they are often overlooked for good practical reasons.[8]

For all of these reasons (and many more) it is not at all easy to demonstrate whether a particular method is effective either for achieving an explicit educational objective or for getting things done in the workplace.

It should also be noted that laboratory-style experiments, in which volunteers are placed artificially into different learning situations, may produce scientifically 'clean' results but these may not be relevant to the real world. For example, small group, problem-based learning (*see* p. 179) has been shown in the laboratory to increase students' ability in the kind of problem solving that can be assessed via formal, reproducible psychometric testing. However, this skill has also been shown to correlate poorly with the ability to solve problems in the real world![5]

In general, the younger the learner and the more precise the competence, the more generalisable are the results of experimental studies. Thus the 'educational laboratory' may be a very good place to test different ways of teaching five-year-olds to read or count, but it is less suitable for evaluating the teaching of clinical problem solving to doctors in training.

The remainder of this chapter describes some 'classic' research studies on the evaluation of small group methods, some of which occurred in the experimental laboratory and some in real-life academic or workplace settings. You may feel, like us, that together these studies amount to a fair body of evidence in favour of small group work in particular situations, but we shall return to their methodological limitations (many of which are unavoidable) at the end of the chapter.

Incidentally, Anna Donald and her team subsequently undertook a comparative study in which Anna delivered traditional lecture-style seminars while one of her colleagues (who was initially somewhat sceptical about the new teaching methods) delivered the small group, problem-based curriculum. Medical students were allocated randomly to the two groups (although randomisation was not concealed, and it was probably theoretically possible for a student to change their allocation). The results confirmed the superiority of the small group methods in terms of popularity with students and examination success.[9]

Studies of the effectiveness of small group, problem-based learning

Most of the evidence on problem-based learning (PBL) (*see* p. 179) in educational settings comes from medical schools in Canada and the USA. PBL was first introduced at McMaster University in Ontario, Canada,[10] and quickly spread to Harvard Medical School.[11] Professor John Bligh is a strong advocate of PBL as well as being one of its fiercest critics, and he has written a brief summary of the pros and cons of the method.[6] The evidence that follows is based on Bligh's summary, together with a review of the literature by Albanese and Mitchell[12] and (most heavily) on a formal meta-analysis of 35 primary studies of PBL in medical education by Vernon and Blake.[13]

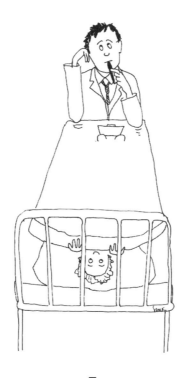

▼

Problem-based learning.

Vernon and Blake defined a study as dealing with PBL if it used small discussion groups, addressed clinical cases, involved collaborative independent study, encouraged hypothetico-deductive reasoning, and included a focus on the small group process as well as on imparting content.[13] They used a comprehensive search strategy and included all research designs that had used some form of quantitative measure of outcome and provided data that allowed the comparison of PBL with more traditional methods on some kind of positive-negative scale (i.e. which attempted to judge whether PBL was *better* rather than just *different*). Studies were included whether they described an entire PBL-based curriculum or a PBL-based course within a more traditional medical curriculum. The authors estimated the methodological limitations of each primary study.

They classified outcome measures in terms of four broad areas, namely student evaluations, academic achievement, academic process (students' perceptions of the methods used) and clinical performance, and where possible they estimated the effect size (i.e. how much better or worse PBL appeared to be).

Vernon and Blake excluded 13 of the 35 studies because no quantitative estimate of effect size could be made for any outcome measure. The remaining 22 studies (on 14 programmes) included five separate designs as follows:

1   *own-control design* – students acted as their own controls (taking a PBL course for one module and a traditional course for a comparable module)
2   *hypothetical-control design* – results obtained for students on a PBL course were compared with hypothetical values representative of traditional methods
3   *static-group design* – students on a largely traditional-style course were asked to volunteer for PBL teaching, and their results were compared with the results of those who had opted to continue on the traditional course
4   *matched static-group design* – as above, but groups were matched for baseline variables thought to be likely to influence results
5   *true experiment* – students (perhaps from a pool of self-selected volunteers) were randomly allocated to PBL or traditional teaching.

The results of the 22 studies are summarised below. (We have not included the quantitative estimates of effect size because the individual studies were methodologically highly heterogeneous, and we believe that the statistical methods used to derive the quantitative estimates are open to criticism.)

Student evaluations

All of the studies in which this outcome was measured showed that students prefer PBL to traditional courses. This supports Bligh's conclusion that PBL is consistently viewed by students as:

- more enjoyable
- more relevant
- more humane
- allowing them to handle uncertainty better than traditional methods.[6]

Academic achievement

Vernon and Blake's analysis suggested that students' scores in medical school examinations were *worse* if teaching was by PBL, although the overall results in this part of the meta-analysis were not statistically significant. The more rigorous research designs (experimental studies), notably the Harvard 'new pathway' programme, generally produced smaller differences between PBL and traditional methods in this outcome. However, there was marked heterogeneity of effect size overall. In other words, large differences between PBL and traditional methods were only seen in some studies, while in others the differences were close to zero or favoured PBL.

Bligh's editorial reflects the continuing uncertainty of the research evidence with regard to academic achievement, but he makes two important observations. First, there is some evidence that knowledge is *retained* for longer in PBL courses, and secondly, the major doubt about PBL in medical school concerns its effectiveness in achieving adequate levels of knowledge in basic science. Bligh tentatively suggests that this particular topic might be better taught by a more teacher-directed method.[6]

Academic process

Only a fraction of the studies in Vernon and Blake's review asked students about the process of learning. Those that did demonstrated consistent results. Students perceived that, compared to traditional courses, PBL courses:

- were less concerned with rote learning and more concerned with understanding or meaning
- used less teacher-selected reading material and more learner-selected material
- made more use of library facilities, on-line searches and academic journals
- made students more confident about their information-seeking skills.

These findings in medical students were confirmed by an independent review of the experimental literature on the psychological basis of PBL.[14] This review supported the notion that PBL improves self-directed learning, and also showed that it increases interest in the subject and (probably) enables the student to transfer concepts to new situations. However, the authors of this overview (confirming their previous work)[5] found no evidence that PBL promotes general, content-free problem-solving skills.

Clinical performance

In general, clinical performance was assessed by observing students' behaviour with real or simulated patients. Overall, Vernon and Blake's review showed that PBL students performed significantly better than traditionally taught students according to this outcome. However, the methods used to define and measure 'good clinical performance' were highly variable and, Vernon and Blake suggest, sometimes of dubious validity.

Another (unpublished) study relevant to clinical performance (discussed by Vernon and Blake but not included in this meta-analysis) was the Harvard 'new pathway' study in which students randomised to PBL or traditional teaching were assessed with regard to five 'skills relating to patients', namely empathy, patient-centredness, comfort with emotion, communication skills and data collection. PBL students outperformed controls on all of these variables, but meaningful comparisons were precluded by the low rate of participation of control students in the evaluation process.[13]

Overall, therefore, there is certainly no evidence that medical students taught by PBL are clinically *less* competent than traditionally taught students, but the evidence from experimental and other trial studies amassed so far falls short of proving that they are *more* competent. We should note, in passing, the widely cited study published in the *Canadian Medical Association Journal* which compared graduates of McMaster University (taught by PBL) and those of a traditional medical school (taught largely by means of 'talk and chalk').[15] There was a statistically significant difference (favouring the McMaster group) in the speed with which these cohorts became out of date in their clinical performance. However, this study was not a randomised controlled trial, it only addressed a single aspect of clinical performance (treatment of hypertension), it examined what doctors said they did rather than what they actually did, and the findings have not been replicated.

In summary, PBL in medical schools has been extensively evaluated, but the vast majority of studies are of non-randomised design and, as such, their conclusions should be viewed with caution. It would appear that PBL produces more satisfied students who may perform slightly less well in traditional examinations (but may retain their knowledge for longer). Tests of clinical competence and humanism probably favour PBL and – lest we forget – no comparative study published to date has looked at the impact on quality of care provided for patients!

Studies of the knowledge required of the facilitator

The practicalities of supporting students in small group PBL can be challenging. Because students define their own learning needs, they frequently stray on to topics in which the facilitator is not an expert. Two studies, both in undergraduate medical schools in the USA,[16,17] were undertaken in order to determine how much this matters (if at all).

Both studies found that students whose small groups had been led by experts in the subject showed the following characteristics compared to those who had been led by non-experts.

- They generated approximately twice as many learning issues per case.
- They generated issues that were more congruent with the learning objectives of the case.
- They spent around twice as much time per case overcoming identified learning deficiencies.
- They showed higher levels of satisfaction with the course.
- They performed significantly better in examinations.

However, another small study of medical undergraduates suggested that in expert-led PBL groups, the facilitator:[18,19]

- takes a more directive role in generating questions
- talks more frequently and for longer than a non-expert facilitator
- spends more time generating learning issues than students spend solving them
- provides direct answers to students' questions, rather than encouraging self-directed learning.

In summary, the published evidence on content expertise is patchy and is derived from a handful of small studies. It suggests that there may be both advantages and disadvantages to including content experts in PBL tutorials, and it also raises questions about how best to optimise the performance of 'expert' PBL facilitators through appropriate training (*see* p. 49).

Conclusion

Small group work in higher education is currently very fashionable. It is widely believed to be more effective than lecture-based methods in achieving deep learning, and there are several theoretical arguments that support this view. In practice, however, the evidence supporting the use of small groups in higher education is patchy, and the widely cited trials comparing and evaluating different educational methods have notable methodological limitations.

We shall probably never 'prove' for certain that small group work has important educational benefits, and we must retain a healthy scepticism about the more ambitious claims that have been made for it. Nevertheless, the accumulated evidence suggests that small group work, and particularly small group problem-based learning, has much to offer the adult learner and should be used more widely in educational settings.

References

1   Norman GR and Schmidt HG (1992) The psychological process of problem-based learning: a review of the evidence. *Acad Med.* **67**: 557–67.

2   Marton F (1997) *The Experience of Learning* (2e). Scottish Academic Press, Edinburgh.

3   Engel C, Vysohlid J and Vodoratski VA (1990) *Continuing Education for Change.* WHO, Geneva.

4   Kolb DA (1993) The process of experiential learning. In: M Thorpe, R Edwards and A Hanson (eds) *Culture and Processes of Adult Learning.* Routledge, London.

5   Norman GR (1988) Problem-solving skills, solving problems, and problem-based learning. *Med Educ.* **22**: 279–86.

6   Bligh J (1995) Problem-based, small group learning. *BMJ.* **311**: 342–3.

7   Neufield VR, Woodward CA and McLeod SM (1989) The McMaster MD programme: a case study in renewal in medical education. *Acad Med.* **64**: 423–32.

8   Cryer P and Elton L (1998) *Conducting Small-Scale Research into Teaching and Learning in Higher Education. Resource Material for Module A. Course text for Postgraduate Diploma in Higher Education Research and Development.* University College London, London.

9   Donald A (2000) *Public health teaching for undergraduate medical students: improving outcomes.* Paper presented at *Teaching and Learning: the way ahead,* UCL, 27 March 2000.

10 Neufield VR, Woodward CA and McLeod SM (1989) The McMaster MD programme: a case study in renewal in medical education. *Acad Med.* **64**: 423–32.

11 Moore GT, Block SD, Style CB and Mitchell R (1994) The influence of the new pathway curriculum on Harvard medical students. *Acad Med.* **69**: 983–9.

12 Albanese MA and Mitchell S (1993) Problem-based learning: a review of the literature on its outcomes and implementation issues. *Acad Med.* **68**: 52–81.

13 Vernon DTA and Blake RL (1993) Does problem-based learning work? A meta-analysis of evaluative research. *Acad Med.* **68**: 550–63.

14 Norman GR and Schmidt HG (1992) The psychological basis of problem-based learning: a review of the evidence. *Acad Med.* **67**: 557–65.

15 Shin JH, Haynes RB and Johnston ME (1993) Effect of problem-based, self-directed undergraduate education on life-long learning. *Can Med Assoc J.* **148**: 969–76.

16 Eagle CJ, Harasym PH and Mandin H (1992) Effects of facilitators with case expertise on problem-based learning issues. *Acad Med.* **67**: 465–9.

17 Davis WK, Nairn R, Paine ME, Anderson RM and Oh MS (1992) Effects of expert and non-expert facilitators on the small-group process and on student performance. *Acad Med.* **67**: 470–4.

18 Wilkerson L, Hafler JP and Liu PA (1991) A case study of student-directed discussion in four problem-based facilitatorial groups. In: Research in Medical Education. Proceedings of the Thirteenth Annual Conference. *Acad Med.* **66** (**Supplement**).

19 Silver M and Wilkerson LA (1991) Effects of facilitators with subject expertise on the problem-based facilitatorial. *Acad Med.* **66**: 298–300.

12

A case study of the use of small groups in postgraduate education: teaching evidence-based healthcare

> *Like dreams, statistics are a form of wish fulfilment.*
> Jean Baudrillard, *Cool Memories*

Background[1]

Much of the progress made in healthcare since the late 1980s can be attributed to the rise in popularity of the 'evidence-based' approach, which states that decisions about tests and treatments should be made on the basis of mathematical estimates of their respective risks and benefits for the patient. These estimates, in turn, should be derived from a rigorous and thorough assessment of the research literature and the incorporation of all relevant values. The increasing recognition that it is also important to integrate the patient's perspective in the decision-making process is another challenge, and is enriching this evidential approach to healthcare management at the individual patient level.[2] Thus the competent clinician is no longer one who has 'the facts' at his or her fingertips, but rather one who knows how to access, prioritise and evaluate an immense and rapidly changing body of knowledge and incorporate the relevant findings with the values and preferences of the patient and society.

Although the evidence-based approach has been welcomed by many clinicians, especially the more academic ones,[3] considerable cultural resistance has been apparent in some circles.[4] Clinical decisions have traditionally been shrouded in mystique and supported by the 'priestly authority' of the senior doctor, rather than being open, defensible, reproducible and shared. It has been a major challenge to get the principles of evidence-based healthcare out of the academic textbook and into the clinic, the operating-theatre and (most difficult of all) the everyday vocabulary of managers, commissioners and purchasers.

Here is an extract from one of the worksheets used in the Second UK Workshop on *Teaching Evidence-Based Health Care*, held at University College London Medical School in February 1996:

> *Read the clinical scenario [about a patient aged 18 months with a single febrile convulsion] and the attached case–control study on the long-term prognosis after febrile seizure in infants. Decide whether and to what extent a single uncomplicated febrile seizure increases the risk of subsequent epilepsy and using a role play or other appropriate teaching techniques, decide how you would convey this information to the child's parents.*

In this and other clinical problems, the 'evidence-based' practitioner must take on aspects of the discipline which do not come naturally and in which he or she was not originally trained. The non-numerate must gain some grasp of statistics, whereas those who like to add up figures must learn to ask where those figures have come from and to apply them to individual circumstances. Clinicians who make decisions on the basis of precise statistical likelihoods must, if they are to share decision making with a truly informed patient, find a way of expressing complex concepts using jargon-free terminology and incorporating patient preferences into their probability trees. In order to achieve sustained behaviour change in fields outside the practitioner's immediate area of expertise, issues such as confidence building, teamwork and intellectual initiative must not be treated as peripheral to the course content.[5]

Methods

It was for all of these reasons that the team at University College London chose to follow the example first set by the McMaster Medical School, Canada,[6] and brought to the UK by Professor Sackett's team in Oxford,[7] and to use small group methods to support delegates in acquiring (and learning how to teach) these multidimensional skills.

We were initially sceptical about replacing the traditional lecture-based conference format with a largely blank timetable, in which delegates' first task was to sit down in groups of eight (with two non-directive facilitators) and decide first what they needed to know and secondly, how they were going to learn it. We provided each group with little more than a seminar room and a flipchart. However, by day two of the six-day workshop, eminent professors were happily engrossed in 'pretending to be medical students not understanding likelihood ratios', senior nurses and geriatricians were role-playing stroke patients and the managers charged with rehabilitating them, and a group of public health physicians were, within the safety of their group, staging a mock press conference to assuage public anxiety about the safety of measles–mumps–rubella vaccine.

The delegates, who derived these diverse teaching scenarios from their own real-life experiences, were required simultaneously to consider the artificial situation they had created ('you are medical students; I am teaching you about likelihood ratios') and the metasituation ('I am someone who is learning to teach; how could I do this more effectively?'). Group members each had an allocated role to play in the simulated teaching scenario, but they and the facilitators could, at any stage, call a 'time-out' (*see* Chapter 4, p. 58) and comment on the metasituation.

Over the years, a tradition has arisen for a variety of 'sideshows', some planned and some spontaneous, which greatly enlivens the workshops. Seminars on statistics and demonstrations of computer software packages and electronic databases provide the opportunity for delegates to work on specific areas of knowledge and skills. In addition, we hold around four plenary sessions during the week, in which we invite external speakers who are eminent in their field to discuss the theoretical principles of group work, teaching and evidence-based practice.

The facilitators in these workshops work in pairs, and each pair of facilitators is placed in a 'buddy group' with three other pairs of facilitators. The buddy group meets daily for about an hour to discuss problems of both process and content and to provide mutual support in what is often an emotionally taxing week. Of course, the buddy group develops its own group identity and undergoes a process of forming, storming, norming and so on in which desirable behaviours are hopefully modelled by more experienced members and serve as learning experiences for the others.

Evaluation

We have been holding 'training the trainers' workshops at University College London (UCL) since 1996 and in Wales since 1997. In total, around 650 delegates have attended these courses. Our approach to evaluation has evolved over the years and is something of a compromise between what we would like to find out and the limits that are set by our time and resources. In addition to administrative aspects, we have sought to address the following six questions.

1   Did the delegates enjoy the workshop and feel it was worthwhile?
2   Did the groups meet the objectives they defined in the first session, and were these sufficiently compatible with individuals' personal objectives?

3   How did the group facilitators perform, and were they appropriately selected and trained?
4   Were non-group activities (plenaries, demonstrations and *ad hoc* sessions) appropriate and worthwhile?
5   Did individuals change their behaviour as a result of attending the workshop and, in particular, did they begin to introduce the principles of evidence-based practice to their home institutions?
6   What was the impact of the workshop on group facilitators?

Satisfaction

Assessment of 'satisfaction' variables using both questionnaires and the nominal group process described in Chapter 19 (*see* p. 305) has been consistently positive throughout all of the workshops. Of particular note is the finding that delegates almost unanimously agreed that the workshop represented 'a good use of the time'.

Group objectives

We made it a principle that evaluations held within a group (*see* pp. 150–1) should not be revealed to the course organisers or form part of the official report. However, feedback from facilitators in buddy groups and via diaries (see below) suggests that groups generally perform well and meet their objectives.

Facilitator performance

We seek information on the performance of the group facilitators, both through free text responses on the individual evaluation questionnaire and by inviting confidential feedback to the course organiser. In addition, we ask the group as a whole to complete the closed-response questionnaire shown in Box 12.1. The aggregated results from the 1999 workshop are shown for information.

Box 12.1:

Facilitator ——— (name)	Has very good knowledge of EBHC	Has fairly good knowledge of EBHC	No view either way *or* group divided	Has fairly poor knowledge of EBHC	Has very poor knowledge of EBHC
	••••••••••	••••••••	•	•	
	Has very good facilitation skills	Has fairly good facilitation skills	No view either way *or* group divided	Has fairly poor facilitation skills	Has very poor facilitation skills
	•••••••••••	••••	•••	••	
	Our group would definitely want this facilitator again	Our group would probably want this facilitator again	No view either way *or* group divided	Our group would probably not want this facilitator again	Our group would definitely not want this facilitator again
	••••••••••• ••	••••		••	•
	Our facilitators worked very well as a pair	Our facilitators worked fairly well as a pair	No view either way	Our facilitators worked fairly poorly as a pair	Our facilitators worked very poorly as a pair
	•••••••	•		••	

EBHC, evidence-based healthcare.

Non-group activities

Plenary sessions on statistics and other 'sideshows' tend to be viewed as very helpful by some delegates and as not at all helpful by others, depending on their own learning needs and styles. Spontaneous *ad hoc* sessions organised by the delegates themselves have, as might be imagined, been of variable quality and drawn mixed evaluations, but at most workshops at least one such session has been evaluated as outstanding.

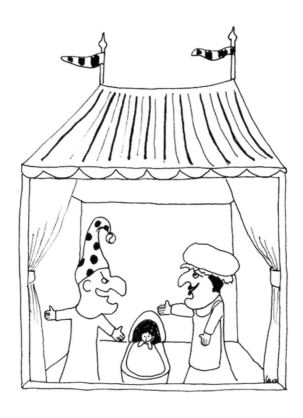

▼

A variety of sideshows greatly enlivens the workshops.

Impact on behaviour

The responses to questionnaires issued before the first UCL workshop revealed that, for many delegates, implementation of evidence-based medicine at their home institutions was limited as much by lack of time, information technology skills, 'political acceptance' and confidence as by lack of knowledge. A questionnaire issued immediately after the workshop (with a response rate of 88%) showed that, despite these barriers, 40% of the 88 delegates intended to introduce new teaching programmes in clinical schools, health authorities or NHS trusts, and of these, all but one planned to use small group, problem-based learning in substantial areas of the curriculum.

An independent evaluation by an external consultant using telephone interviews two years after the first UCL workshop (with a response rate of 57%)[8] suggested that many of the delegates had indeed become innovators in the field of evidence-based practice. Examples of major changes in organisational strategy, purchase (and use) of dedicated computer equipment for evidence-based healthcare at an organisation-wide level, innovations in curriculum development, and the establishment of systematic training programmes for staff were commonly cited. However, as the author of this report stated, the individuals who attended this early workshop (which was heavily oversubscribed) were probably 'movers and shakers' who might have initiated these changes anyway. She felt that it was impossible to determine the impact of the workshop itself, although many delegates felt that it had been a seminal experience. Another external evaluation conducted 10 months after one of the courses in Wales revealed that the educational impact of the course was very high, and that the majority of participants felt they understood the principle of basing their practice on sound evidence. However, they did report that their service environment often made it extremely difficult to put their theory into practice.[9]

Impact on facilitators

These workshops are one of the most demanding tasks that a small group facilitator can face. They are faced with the intricacies of a small group process, coupled with an intense week of work for most participants as they face the learning curves of both biostatistics and an examination of their teaching techniques at close quarters. There are inevitable conflicts, and one way of capturing the process from the tutor's perspective is to ask them to keep a diary after every group section and to share the non-confidential aspects of this for systematic analysis. Using this method, the inherent tensions in these courses were demonstrated. A conflict existed between the variation in learning cultures exhibited by the delegates, and the effect that this has on processes.

For example, there was tension between the reductionist approach of biomedicine and the more qualitative research ethos of the applied and 'caring' disciplines such as nursing. There was also a conflict between the goal of 'learning' about applied healthcare biostatistics (content) and the ability to leave the course with the skills to teach others (process).[10] The facilitators have to be able to tread this tightrope.

It could be argued that the organisers of the evidence-based healthcare workshops should take responsibility for demonstrating a worthwhile improvement in patient care as a result of the training they offer. Although we fully acknowledge the need for hard, patient-relevant outcomes to be demonstrated, we do not feel it is either feasible or affordable for the organisers of educational courses to address the 'bottom line' in this way. Youll has argued that responsibility for evaluation should occur at four different levels,[8] as shown in Table 12.1.

Table 12.1:   Levels at which a training workshop on evidence-based practice could be evaluated (based on Youll)[8]

Descriptor	Evaluation question	Evaluation method	Responsibility for addressing this question
Level 1: The course as an educational opportunity	'Did we provide adequate educational resources and appropriately trained facilitators?'	Assessment of satisfaction by questionnaire	Course organiser
Level 2: The course as a learning experience	'Did people's knowledge, understanding, motivation and attitudes change?'	Assessment of knowledge, beliefs and attitudes by questionnaire	Course organiser
Level 3: The course as a vehicle for behaviour change in health professionals	'Did clinical practice improve?'	Process measures of clinical practice (e.g. extent to which practitioner follows a guideline)	Individual learner and/or continuing professional education sponsor
Level 4: The course as an intervention to improve overall patient care in an organisation	'Were patients better off?'	Outcome measures in terms of patient health and quality of life (e.g. rates of hysterectomy, teenage pregnancy, stroke, etc.)	Training officer and/or clinical governance lead in the organisation

Developing the workshops

The UK workshops on teaching evidence-based healthcare,[7,11] which have so far been held in Oxford, London, Cardiff, Edinburgh and Newcastle, like their counterparts in North America have been extremely popular and generally well evaluated. Their success can be partly attributed to the sound learning methods, and to the well-described positive effect of small group work on affective dimensions of learning (in a nutshell, a one-week workshop based on group work is great fun!).

However, demand for training in evidence-based healthcare in recent years has been greatly enhanced by the political climate in the UK (and beyond). Since 1999, for example, health professionals and managers in the UK National Health Service (NHS) have had a contractual duty of 'clinical governance' (i.e. they can be held personally accountable for the quality of care received by patients). Training budgets in public sector healthcare must be seen to be spent on promoting evidence-based practice and other 'quality'

initiatives. Furthermore, many NHS professionals can potentially reap financial rewards (or incur penalties) for providing services that are more (or less)
congruent with the best current research evidence.

In one respect, therefore, the success of the 'teaching evidence-based
healthcare' workshops is guaranteed, at least in the foreseeable future. At the
time of writing, the numbers of applications continue to exceed the places
available by a substantial amount. Speaking for the workshops we ourselves
are involved in, we have initiated a strategy for continuous quality improvement to ensure that the content and style of the workshops are relevant to the
needs of the delegates. This strategy includes the following:

1   formal evaluation of each workshop using the methods described above,
    with production of a written evaluation report that is intended mainly for
    internal use
2   an 'away-day' for course organisers and selected facilitators, held several
    weeks after the workshop, to allow reflection on the evaluation report
    and informal feedback, and to plan changes to administrative arrange-
    ments, staff training, recruitment, group allocation, IT support and the
    programme itself. One important strategic change which we have
    successfully made was to increase the proportion of non-medical delegates
    at these workshops – it has risen from under 10% in 1996 to over 50% in
    2000 (London figures)
3   a rolling programme of training and support for facilitators, including an
    annual two-day training workshop focusing mainly on facilitation and
    troubleshooting techniques, but also including content (e.g. statistics) if
    requested
4   development of a programme of 'second-level' workshops in response
    to feedback from delegates. Some of the more experienced delegates had
    suggested that, having already mastered the key techniques for teaching
    evidence-based healthcare, they were still not adequately equipped to
    implement major changes in clinical practice in their home institutions
    (typically medical or nursing schools, GP practices, hospitals or health
    authorities). They sought additional training in the skills of change man-
    agement, and we have begun to offer such workshops, based on the same
    small group format but facilitated by individuals trained in management
    and organisational behaviour rather than in clinical epidemiology.[12]

Conclusion

This series of workshops, which began in Canada in the late 1980s, is one
of the most striking waves of events in adult medical education in recent
years. It was instrumental in shifting the paradigm for continuing medical

education away from unidisciplinary, didactic lectures to small group, problem-based learning. It pre-dated and may have influenced the change in policy for funding continuing professional development in general practice away from attendance at educational lectures and towards multidisciplinary professional and practice development plans.[13] However, small group, multidisciplinary learning for evidence-based practice is not cheap. The NHS and other organisations struggle to resource this kind of training, especially when cheaper, lecture-based courses are readily available. The survival of these workshops, in common with other similar initiatives, depends on political will and a policy of long-term investment in human resources.

References

1   Greenhalgh T (1997) Workshops for teaching evidence-based practice. *Evidence-Based Med.* **2**: 7–8.

2   Elwyn G, Edwards A and Kinnersley P (1999) Shared decision-making: the neglected second half of the consultation. *Br J Gen Pract.* **49**: 477–82.

3   Lipman T, Rogers S and Elwyn G (1997) Evidence-based medicine in primary care: some views from the Third UK Workshop on Teaching Evidence-Based Medicine. *Evidence-Based Med.* **2**: 133–5.

4   Stradling JR and Davies RJO (1997) The unacceptable face of evidence-based medicine. *J Eval Clin Pract.* **3**: 99–103.

5   Norman GR and Schmidt HG (1992) The psychological basis of problem-based learning: a review of the evidence. *Acad Med.* **67**: 557–65.

6   Neufield VR, Woodward CA and McLeod SM (1989) The McMaster MD programme: a case study in renewal in medical education. *Acad Med.* **64**: 423–32.

7   http://cebm.jr2.ox.ac.uk/docs/workshopsteaching.html

8   Youll P (1997) *Long-term Evaluation of 2nd UK Workshop on Teaching Evidence-based Health Care.* Internal Report to North Thames RHA.

9   Wilby P and Elwyn G (1999) The 'evidence-based' workshop experience: a 10-month follow-up study. *J Interprof Care.* **13**: 190–1.

10   Elwyn G, Rosenberg W, Edwards A *et al.* (2000) Diaries of evidence-based tutors: beyond 'numbers needed to teach'. *J Clin Eval.* (In press.)

11   For further details of the London Workshops on Teaching Evidence-based Health Care *see* http://www.ucl.ac.uk/primcare-popsci/uebpp/ttt.htm

12   For further details of the London Workshops on Managing Change for Effective Clinical Practice *see* http://www.ucl.ac.uk/primcare-popsci/uebpp/chm.htm

13   Elwyn G (1998) Professional and practice development plans for primary care teams. *BMJ.* **317**: 1454–5.

13

The virtual group

Reality leaves a lot to the imagination.
John Lennon, TV interview

Computer-assisted learning

Computer-assisted learning is a major growth industry, with both universities and commercial companies producing self-study materials either on the Internet or on CD-ROM. Distance learning favours the able, motivated, mature and well organised student, but until fairly recently the distance learner was denied many of the most fulfilling aspects of academic study, namely interactive tutorials, seminars, and informal discussions with tutors and fellow students.

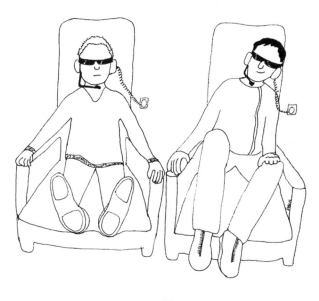

▼

The familiar landmarks of university interaction replaced by virtual alternatives.

As Table 13.1 shows, the role of the computer has changed dramatically over the past 50 years.

Table 13.1:   Changing role of the computer

Date	Role of the computer
1950s	Computer was an adding machine, used mainly for complex and tedious mathematical calculations
1960s	Computer was a filing system, used to store information
1970s	Computer was a library, used to store and access educational and instructional materials
1980s	Computer was a personal assistant, used to facilitate the efficient indexing and retrieval of information
1990s	Computer was a communication channel, used to transmit messages rapidly between individuals
2000s	Computer is a facilitator that can be used to bring individuals together and aid their communication and collaboration in groups

Most of us are comfortable with (and perhaps dependent on) the computer as a powerful calculator or as a store of readily accessible and searchable information. However, many people fail to recognise the enormous potential of this medium for changing the nature of interactions both in education and in the workplace.[1] Lewis Elton, Professor of Higher Education at University College London, has argued that if a student from AD 1300 travelled forward in time to a university in AD 2000, he or she would immediately recognise it as a familiar institution. However, if a student from AD 2000 travelled just 20 years into the future, the familiar landmarks of university interaction (such as the lecture theatre, seminar, debating chamber and perhaps even the student bar) might have all but disappeared and been replaced by 'virtual' alternatives.

Educational programmes based on computer-mediated interaction between tutors and students were, somewhat predictably, first used in computer science courses. Postgraduate business studies courses (notably at the UK's Open University, which now has over 6000 active users on MBA and short courses,[2] and a handful of 'mega-universities' throughout North America and Asia)[3] followed, and examples of virtual learning groups can now be found in almost every academic subject.[4]

Types of virtual group

There are four main underlying technologies that can be used for virtual group work.

Simple email exchange

This is the cheapest and most straightforward way of running a virtual group. Each participant creates a 'nickname' on their personal email server that lists the email addresses of all the other members. Whenever a participant wishes to send a message to the group, they use the 'nickname' rather than individual addresses. If they wish to reply to a communication, they copy it to everyone by means of the 'nickname' (or use the 'reply to all' button).

This form of virtual group is easy to set up, and can be very spontaneous and informal. It is often used to enable the members of a face-to-face group to maintain contact after a course or workshop. We ourselves used this method to keep in touch with one another while writing this book! The problem with simple email is that messages are not threaded (*see* Box 13.2, p. 213), the on-screen environment is very basic (e.g. there are no pictures or colour) and there are no mechanisms for making the interaction more sophisticated (*see* section on specialised software below). In addition, the rapid response facility (it only takes a second to press the 'reply' button) can make the more impulsive participant send messages which they later regret.

Exchange of email via list server

In this method, a central server automatically distributes email messages to all members on the list. Many such lists are co-ordinated through the central academic mail server in the UK known as mailbase.ac.uk. These groups have open membership (i.e. anyone who fulfils the entry criteria may join up, and anyone may leave). Some examples of centrally run academic mailing lists, and details of how to join, are given at the end of this chapter.

Membership of academic mailing lists tends to fluctuate considerably. Some lists have a few dozen members, while others have over a thousand. Some have a designated moderator, but many do not, and both the amount and the quality of interaction vary with different lists. You can join one of the above lists to get a flavour of this type of virtual group work without having to post any messages yourself, as no one on the list will know that you have joined unless you send a message. Receiving messages from a list without sending any oneself is known as 'lurking' and, in contrast to face-to-face group work, nobody seems to mind the presence of silent lurkers!

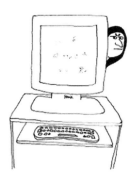

▼

Nobody seems to mind the presence of silent lurkers.

Specialised group software

There are several commercial packages available for running virtual groups. Most such packages are run via a website on the Internet to which group members log on via a personal password. The advantages of using dedicated software rather than simple email include the following.

- The screen can be customised in a similar manner to a web page using colour, icons (on-screen pictures and symbols), an institutional logo, and so on. If the on-screen environment is well designed, the virtual group looks and feels more professional and 'corporate' than is the case with email exchange, but note that the overuse of customisation features will make the site appear tacky and commercial (for further useful advice on creating a suitable on-screen environment for group work, see Giles and Salmon's paper).[5]
- Messages are systematically sorted ('threaded') and indexed automatically.
- On-line 'chat' (synchronous communication; *see* p. 212) is often possible.
- Participants can create their own web pages and other personalised materials (*see* p. 208).
- Additional features can be incorporated, such as on-screen evaluation questionnaires.
- Many packages offer the facility for creating an entire on-line curriculum, of which virtual group work constitutes one feature.

The disadvantages of using commercial group software packages include the following:

- price
- complexity
- the need for training and 'helpdesk' support for participants.

The characteristics of some of the commoner groupware packages are summarised in Table 13.2 (*see* p. 208).

Video-conferencing

The use of video links is increasingly common in both education (for lectures, seminars and specialist demonstrations, e.g. post-mortems) and management (for meetings within or between organisations). Several researchers have studied the effect of video-conferencing on the group process.[6-8] All of these authors emphasise both the time and scale advantages of video-conferencing and the potential for developing innovative techniques for teaching and decision making. Group work in a video-conferencing environment has the following well-documented features compared to face-to-face interaction.

- More time needs to be put into planning and preparation.
- Technical problems can and do occur – with a variable effect on the group process and individual members (some become diverted into 'fixing' the technology, while others 'switch off' or become frustrated).
- The experience is more mentally demanding as participants must concentrate simultaneously on the content of the meeting, the visual material, the home site and the remote site.
- Non-verbal cues are less easily detected (see below), and all parties need to be more proactive in giving and seeking cues.
- Impromptu digressions or expansions (e.g. drawing a diagram on a flip chart) are more difficult to accommodate.
- In video-conferenced teaching situations, the tutor is less able (for example) to 'look over a student's shoulder' to see that he or she has grasped a concept. Hence the onus tends to be more on students to request individual help rather than on the tutor to offer it.

Audio-conferencing

In most developed countries, anyone with a telephone can arrange a multi-user 'conference call' by prearranging it with a central switchboard run by a major telephone company. Participants in the conference are given a special number to call at a particular time and, usually guided by one of the callers who acts as a chairperson, they take turns in speaking. Audio-conferencing is much easier and cheaper than video-conferencing. Clearly it has the disadvantage of a complete absence of visual cues, but it does offer a low-technology alternative to video-conferencing or a face-to-face meeting. Audio-conferencing may be particularly appropriate if:

- the task to be addressed is simple and not dependent on visual aids
- the number of participants in the group is less than five
- everyone is an active participant – audio groups have a low tolerance of 'lurkers'
- all participants have the same mother tongue (or are highly fluent in the language used)
- the chairperson is experienced in this medium.

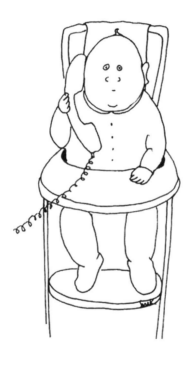

▼

Anyone with a telephone can arrange a multi-user 'conference call'.

What is different about virtual groups?

Virtual groups should not be thought of as simply another technique (comparable with, for example, seminars or buzz groups; *see* Table 1.1, p. 6), but rather as an entirely new *context* within which any of the techniques listed in Chapter 5 (*see* pp. 77–93) might be tried (perhaps with modification).[9] As we emphasised in Chapter 2, the culture and context of the group are an extremely important determinant of the interaction in the group, and we should consider carefully the new learning culture created by computer technology.

The virtual group process differs crucially from its face-to-face equivalent in the following six areas:

- dependence on technology
- absence of non-verbal cues
- place of interaction
- timing of interaction
- facility for private communication
- recording of the group process.

Dependence on technology

There are obviously some technological prerequisites for virtual group work. Each member must have:

- a personal computer (or terminal) that is able to run the software (if any) used for the group work
- a modem or other connection with the Internet.

In addition, if specialised software is used (*see* Table 13.2), there must be a central server to store and organise the messages, and if a video link is required it must be established and maintained. The cost of hardware and software, and of telephone line charges where applicable, often proves to be a more significant barrier to participation than the organisers of the project initially assumed.[9] The amount of training that is needed for a person to become confident in the use of specialised software packages should not be underestimated.[1,10] Research at Duke University in the USA found that students spent most of their first term getting to grips with the technology, and that this substantially reduced the amount of coursework they were able to cover.[11]

Hillman and colleagues from the Open University Business School have demonstrated that students on on-line distance learning courses do not learn all of the essential skills at the outset of the course.[12] Rather, they employ 'just-in-time learning' (i.e. most of them make no attempt to get to grips with a feature of the software until they actually need to use that feature).[2] Salmon has proposed a five-stage model of the way in which students acquire competence in computer-based interactive learning. These stages are summarised in Figure 13.1.

The notion of 'just-in-time learning' has important implications for the design of induction and training courses to prepare participants for virtual group work. Specifically, too much 'upfront' training may be neither popular

Table 13.2:   'Groupware': commercial software packages for virtual group work

Package	Key features	Website for further details
WebCT	Designed and supported by the Department of Computer Science at the University of British Columbia, Canada, World-wide, probably the most widely used package for educational courses. Highly customisable, with a wide range of optional features for delivering on-line courses. End user requires a minimum of hardware. Twenty-four-hour technical support from the University of British Columbia helpdesk. Good value for money	http://www.webct.com/
First Class	Designed predominantly for computer-mediated conferencing (CMC), and used mainly outside the university setting for conferencing and continuing professional development	http://serverwatch.internet.com/ webserver-fcis.html
Lotus Notes	Another popular package for both academic and commercial group work	http://www.lotus.com/home.nsf/ welcome/lotusnotes

nor effective. However, the Open University's research findings relate to students who do all their learning on-line. Preliminary data from the new virtual MSc course in Primary Health Care at University College London, in which students attend an intensive on-site summer school for training in the use of the webCT software, suggests that using this method, sufficient skills can be acquired to enable students to cope technically with all aspects of the course from the outset.

Absence of non-verbal cues

As Figure 13.1 shows, the acquisition of appropriate technology is a relatively superficial hurdle on the way towards achieving effective group work in a virtual environment.[13] The entire *culture* of virtual communication is profoundly different from face-to-face interaction.[14] In a conventional face-to-face group, participants are essentially using the same communication skills they learned at mother's knee, namely facial expressions such as smiling or frowning, changes in verbal emphasis or tone of voice, hand gestures, and the subtle use of eye contact. Although many aspects of face-to-face group work must be learned and agreed as 'ground rules' (*see* p. 102), the basic currency of communication does not need to be relearned.

In contrast, the participants in a virtual group must, in addition to becoming technically adept in using the software, learn a host of different cues and

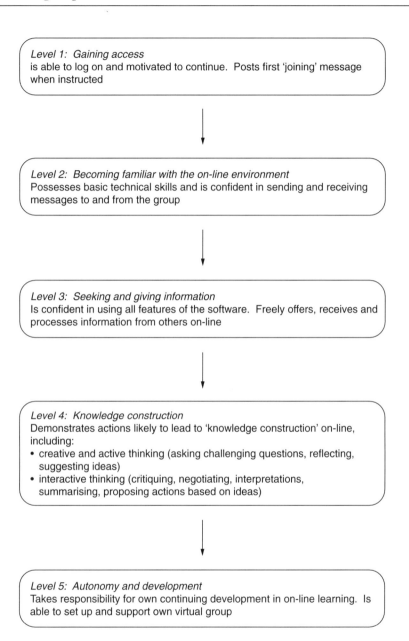

Figure 13.1: Stages in the development of competence in virtual group work (based on Salmon's five-stage model for training the trainers).[13]

techniques for communication. They cannot see from 'body language' whether their fellow participants are receptive, supportive, bored, hostile or inattentive. If you post a message in a virtual group, you do not know for certain when (or if) people will read what you have written. McMahon distinguished between students who 'lose themselves' and those who 'find themselves' in the virtual environment,[15] and Salmon observed similarly that whereas some students perceived their virtual group to be part of a warm, friendly and supportive on-line community ('in here'), others regarded themselves as facing a whole sea of others ('out there').[16] It would appear that the virtual group can be an emotionally barren and socially alien environment compared to the cosiness of face-to-face interaction – at least until the participant is familiar with the new culture. Table 13.3 suggests some virtual equivalents of traditional non-verbal cues.

Table 13.3:   Suggestions for virtual substitutes for non-verbal cues in group work

Traditional non-verbal cue	Usual interpretation of this behaviour	Indicator of similar emotional response in virtual group
Smiling, positive facial expression, leaning forward	Support, warmth, empathy, interest	Explicit postings (e.g. 'Well said' or 'I agree') which have been termed 'say-writing'[17] or 'emoticons'[18] (e.g. ^5 = high five (((name))) = hug)
'Secret' body language between two members (e.g. winking, eye contact)	Empathy, peer support (especially when there is aggression or negative feedback from a third party)	Private email message
Laughter or other emotional 'releases'	Relief of tension	Verbal humour or emoticons[18] (e.g. ;-) = wink :-0 = surprise :-D = laugh)
Sitting outside the circle group members; using 'closed' body language	Withdrawal from the group	Reduction in frequency of postings from that member or emoticons (see below)
Yawning	Boredom (especially if displayed by several members	Few or no responses on this topic from other group members, or emoticons[18] (e.g. |-0 = yawn :-(= frown/sad)
Aggressive gestures accompanying speech (e.g. standing up, table thumping)	Attempt to convey strong emotion (e.g. anger)	Use of capital letters (e.g. 'DON'T FLY OFF THE HANDLE – I WAS ONLY TRYING TO HELP') or emoticon (e.g. :-> = shouting)
Emphatic gestures accompanying speech (e.g. hand waving, drawing on pipe)	Drawing attention to key words or phrases	Use of asterisks around the key words (e.g. 'I think we should discuss the *sexual* implications of this case')

Place of interaction

A virtual group can have members anywhere in the world. Apart from the obvious liberation from the tedium of travel, this enhances the potential for bringing together people from very different backgrounds. Members of a virtual group may have far fewer shared assumptions and values, and they may even speak different languages (*see* example in Box 13.1). The additional burden that this creates for both the participants and the facilitator is often overlooked in the face of the more immediate and obvious challenges of computer-based interaction.

Box 13.1:   Example of cultural and linguistic difficulties in a virtual small group

Sharon *(from England)*	I enjoyed the set chapter on the role of the primary healthcare team in the prevention of disease. It strikes me that PCGs are in a unique position to take a lead in preventive healthcare, but I don't think this could happen unless PCGs are allowed protected time and resources for this. I think NICE should come up with some recommendations.
Denis *(from the USA)*	Surely prevention is the government's job, and they should be able to take over television programmes and put articles in the papers. No one is going to pay you for sitting them down and telling them not to smoke, drink, etc.
Sophia *(from Greece)*	I am not fully understanding this discussion. I am not sure what you say is nice for prevention.
Sharon	Sorry. 'NICE' stands for National Institute for Clinical Excellence. It's an official UK watchdog on the quality and cost of health technologies, especially drug therapies.
Mohammed *(from Pakistan)*	I think Sharon is saying that preventive care should be organised by committees of experts in primary care. I can't really comment on how things go in the UK, but I do know that in rural Pakistan it's hard to ignore factors like poor water quality, high rates of HIV in prostitutes, and the shameless advertising by tobacco companies to the poorest sectors of society. These are all crucial prevention issues, and they must also be relevant to the rest of the world.
Denis	I agree these issues are important for society as a whole. But I don't understand why individual doctors should get involved in them. As an individual doctor you should be doing your best for the patient in front of you.

The example shown in Box 13.1 demonstrates that cultural differences can offer a potentially rich learning experience, as participants must quickly recognise the contextual nature of their own perspective and acknowledge the existence of very different ways of looking at the problem. However, such cross-cultural exchanges are hard work and require careful facilitation. In the virtual MSc in primary healthcare at University College London,[19] students are asked to prepare a personal web page that describes their own professional background as well as the religious, socio-economic and political context of the country or region where they practise. Fellow students can then interpret apparently bizarre or inappropriate comments in the light of this background information.

Timing of interaction

There are two fundamental ways in which people can interact by computer:

- *synchronous (real time) interaction* – in which everyone logs on at the same time and sees the letters on the screen as they are typed in by different participants. This method, usually referred to as 'chat', is commonly employed for recreational purposes, but is relatively little used in official courses
- *asynchronous interaction* – in which members of the group each log in at their own convenience, check for new contributions from their fellow participants, and post their own new messages for others to see.

Asynchronous interaction has a number of theoretical advantages, which research is now beginning to confirm in practice. First, the participants are freed of temporal as well as geographical constraints. Busy professionals with unpredictable workloads (notably doctors and business executives) and those with domestic or other commitments can, if they wish, do their 'group work' at a time that other members of the group would find distinctly antisocial.

Secondly, and perhaps more significantly, the virtual group process allows more *reflection* than does face-to-face interaction. Participants can take as much time as they wish to consider the contribution of another group member and formulate their response. The less able or confident member can draft a response and reflect on it before sending it to the rest of the group. People who feel that they 'never get a word in edgeways' can create additional opportunities to participate by logging on more frequently. Conversely, individuals with a tendency to make hasty comments that they later regret can construct a response but delay sending it until the following day, when a more measured contribution may have occurred to them.

Finally, because contributions are 'threaded' (i.e. responses are automatically linked to the comment to which they pertain, rather than to the last comment made by any group member), asynchronous communication allows discussion to proceed in a non-linear manner. For example, consider the asynchronous discussion shown in Box 13.2, which follows a reading task and assignment on the rationing of healthcare. The messages can either be read in temporal sequence as shown here, or the reader can follow the two threads separately by selecting the 'next in thread' icon at the end of each message.

Box 13.2:   Example of asynchronous group discussion showing two separate conversation threads

Sally	*Thread: Burke and Blake [1]* What did everyone else think of the chapter by Burke and Blake on rationing healthcare? I didn't feel it covered the ethical dimension at all.
James	*Thread: Alzheimer's disease [1]* My grandmother suffers from Alzheimer's disease, and she's been told that she can't have a new medication because it's too expensive, even though there's good evidence that it prevents progression. It's rationing by age, not by need, if you ask me.
Mohammed	*Thread: Burke and Blake [2]* I agree, Sally. I thought these guys were only concerned with the economics of rationing and explaining quality-adjusted life years as if these were completely unproblematic.
Simon	*Thread: Burke and Blake [3]* That's not entirely true. Look at the bottom of page 351 when they describe two different theoretical approaches to the ethics of healthcare rationing.
Ravina	*Thread: Alzheimer's disease [2]* James, surely it's reasonable to make some rationing decisions on the basis of age. After all, if someone's got a maximum life expectancy of five years, their life is surely worth less than a child who has 70 or 80 years to live for?
Tutor	*Thread: Burke and Blake [4]* There seems to be some controversy about whether Burke and Blake have covered the ethical aspects of healthcare rationing adequately. Would anyone like to suggest what ethical criteria we should use when deciding how to spend limited resources for healthcare? (If you'd like to see a specific example of an ethical dilemma, see James and Ravina's correspondence in the 'Alzheimer's disease' thread.)

The use of threads is one aspect of virtual group work that participants must learn and adhere to, since inadvertently posting a response to one message as a reply to a different message will quickly generate confusion in the group.

We suggest that the lack of visual and other non-verbal cues may have advantages as well as disadvantages. For example, it is not immediately obvious that the person who has made a comment on a bulletin board (email message forum) is black or white, male or female, beautiful or ugly, or speaks with an accent that betrays a particular social class. Some readers may remember how self-consciousness about acne or body size inhibited their contributions to seminars when they were undergraduates. As a more extreme example, one student on an Open University course even admitted in a formal evaluation interview that 'Until I tried working in a virtual group, I didn't realise that women had anything intellectual to offer'![20]

Potential for private interaction in parallel with group work

In face-to-face group work, if the tutor (or another group member) sees someone displaying antisocial behaviour, they can only intervene publicly, or else must wait until the session has finished. In the virtual group situation, it is possible to send a private email either to the disruptive member (thus sparing him or her the embarrassment of a confrontation in front of the whole group) or to another member to offer support or suggest a way of responding.

We ourselves have experienced the (arguably) inappropriate use of private email by dominant members of academic mailing lists who have attempted to 'bully' less experienced members privately rather than share their responses with the list as a whole. However, we have also seen the same technique used very effectively to encourage a reticent member of a mailing list to persevere with a public communication. The use of private email to supplement shared communications is one of many aspects of virtual group work on which very little research has so far been published.

Recording of the group process

Whether the participants like it or not, the electronic medium automatically creates a detailed, permanent and fully indexed record of the entire group process. Individual group members may look back over the contributions that have been made, and remind their fellow participants of messages which were sent several days or weeks previously. Tutors may call attention to particular sequences of communication in order to illustrate lessons about the group process (which may have gone unnoticed at the time as participants focused on content). Whereas video-recording of a face-to-face group fundamentally changes the interaction (because people 'play to camera'), the recording of the virtual group process generally goes unnoticed, creating a potentially rich archive for researchers![12]

Unanswered research questions about the virtual group

Research into virtual learning has, certainly up until the time of writing, lagged behind the technology.[8] Salmon has made some preliminary suggestions about the appropriate theoretical framework for this kind of research.[13] Based on the work of Metz,[9] Wild[10] and Jonassen and colleagues,[21] she argues for a constructivist, learner-centred approach. In other words, the focus should *not* be on conducting experimental studies that compare one system with another in terms of psychometric outcomes defined by the researchers. Rather, it should be on achieving a detailed description of the needs of the learner and defining specific barriers to meeting them in particular real-life learning situations, so as to 'enlighten what we already know about what works and what doesn't work in this area'. This interpretive approach is supported by Cryer and Elton's more general recommendations for conducting small-scale research into teaching and learning in higher education.[22]

We list below some important research questions about the virtual group process that have occurred to us, and we invite readers to contact us with further suggestions for the focus or methods of research in this rapidly advancing field.

Does a virtual group gain from meeting face to face at some stage?

There are many reports of virtual groups that have never met one another (the Open University probably has the largest archive of such groups), and some such groups can clearly function very effectively, especially if the facilitators are properly trained. However, it is common experience for a group to feel 'closer' after a face-to-face meeting. We ourselves feel that the most important aspects of group work are those listed on pp. 5–7 (active participation, a common task, and reflection), and whilst these key features can be nurtured effectively in the face-to-face setting, they can also be promoted on-line. The need for further exploratory research in this area is evident!

What are the specific training, support and resource needs for tutors and facilitators of virtual groups?

Rowntree has emphasised that to support tutors in running virtual groups, their own training and support should be delivered on-line. 'Virtual' training will both model the use of the appropriate medium and also ensure that the tutors are entirely comfortable with on-line methods before they use them with students.[14] However, we do not know what is the best style or technique for such on-line support. Salmon and her colleagues have started to map the research territory in training virtual group facilitators,[13] but there are still many more questions than answers.

What are the barriers to learning in a virtual interactive environment, and how can these barriers be overcome?

As we described on p. 210, the virtual environment can be a barrier to rather than a channel for effective group interaction. The notion that some participants 'lose themselves' and others 'find themselves' in the virtual environment (and perhaps that everyone might eventually find themselves, given the right 'comfort zones')[16] raises many additional questions about the characteristics of participants who succeed in particular on-line contexts.

What is the optimum number of participants in a virtual group, and how frequently should the tutor log on in order to moderate?

Giles and Salmon have suggested (on the basis of their extensive personal experience) that optimum numbers will vary considerably, depending on the purpose of the virtual group. For example, they make the following recommendations:[9]

- *for research and discussion purposes* – between 3 and 20 participants, and moderate frequently
- *for collaborative working* – up to 9 participants, and moderate weekly
- *for debate* – up to 50 list members with around 6 members taking active roles, and moderate twice weekly

- *for support for groups that also meet face to face* – up to 50 participants, and moderate occasionally.

These figures, which are all derived from the Open University Business School on-line courses, provide a useful rule of thumb. However, we suggest that additional, more detailed research is needed in a wider variety of virtual environments to confirm, extend or challenge these estimates.

Academic mailing lists

These include the following:

- *distancelearn-research* – a forum for the wider discussion of research in distance learning, including educational, social, psychological, technical and administrative issues
- *creativity-in-education* – a forum dedicated to creating a community of enquiry across the educational spectrum, sharing creative ideas for facilitating and evaluating good practice, and disseminating information
- *evidence-based-health* – a multidisciplinary discussion group on clinical epidemiology
- *gp-uk* – a forum for general practitioners in the UK
- *quality-management* – a forum for the exchange of ideas and information by researchers and practitioners involved in the field of quality management and continuous improvement practices
- *lis-medical* and *lis-nursing* – two lists established by the Libraries and Information Systems for Medicine and Nursing, respectively, to provide a forum to facilitate discussion by library and information professionals who are involved in these disciplines.

For a full list of academic mailing lists, see the website http://mailbase.ac.uk/

To join one of these lists (in general you do not need to be either an academic or resident in the UK, although some lists have specific entry criteria), send an email to postmaster@mailbase.ac.uk with the following as the only line in the message body:

> Subscribe name-of-list firstname lastname

For example:

> Subscribe evidence-based-health John Smith

You may find that you are quickly inundated with messages that do not interest you after all, in which case you can remove yourself by sending the following message to postmaster:

> Unsubscribe name-of-list

If you want a temporary break from the messages, send this message:

> Suspend mail name-of-list

If you are a member of several lists and wish to take a break from them all (e.g. because you are going on holiday), send this message:

> Suspend mail all

To resume your mail, send the following message:

> Resume mail name-of-list [or all].

References

1   Dillemans R, Lowyck J, Van der Pere G, Claeys C and Elen J (1998) *New Technologies for Learning*. Leuven University Press, Leuven.

2   Salmon G. *Creating New Models for Organisational Learning*. Open University, Milton Keynes. Unpublished paper available on-line on http://oubs.open.ac.uk/gilly

3   Daniel JS (1996) *Mega-Universities and Knowledge Media. Technology Strategies for Higher Education*. Kogan Page, London.

4   Reingold H (1995) *The Virtual Community*. Minerva, London.

5   Giles KE and Salmon G. *Creating and Implementing Successful On-Line Learning Environments: a Practitioner Perspective*. Open University, Milton Keynes. Unpublished paper available on-line on http://oubs.open.ac.uk/gilly

6   Lee M and Thompson R. *Teaching at a Distance: Building a Virtual Learning Environment*. Centre for Computer-Based Learning. Queen's University, Belfast. Unpublished paper available on-line on http://www.jtap.ac.uk

7   Mason R (1994) *Using Communications Media in Open and Flexible Learning*. Kogan Page, London.

8   Jacobs G and Rodgers C (1997) Remote teaching with digital video: a transnational experience. *Br J Educ Technol*. **28**: 292–304.

9   Metz M (1994) Computer-mediated communication: literature review of a new context. *Int Comput Technol*. **2**: 31–49.

10 Wild M (1996) Technology refusal: rationalising the failure of student and beginning teachers to use computers. *Br J Educ Technol*. **27**: 134–43.

11 Mason R (1998) *Global Education*. Routledge, London.

12 Hillman DCA, Willis DJ and Gunawardena CN (1994) Learner–interface interaction in distance education: an extension of contemporary models and strategies for practitioners. *Am J Dist Educ*. **28**: 30–42.

13 Salmon G. *On The Line. Developing Conferencing Within a Distance Learning Management Education Context: Training the Tutors*. Open University, Milton Keynes. Unpublished paper available on-line on http://oubs.open.ac.uk/gilly

14   Rowntree D (1995) Teaching and learning on-line: a correspondence education for the twenty-first century? *Br J Educ Technol.* **26**: 205–15.

15   McMahon H (1993) Distant bubbles. In: R Mason (ed) *Computer Conferencing: the Last Word.* Beach Holme, Victoria, British Colombia.

16   Salmon G (2000) *E-moderating: a Guide to Tutoring and Mentoring On-Line.* Kogan Page, London.

17   Mason R (1993) Written interactions. In: R Mason (ed) *Computer Conferencing: the Last Word.* Beech Holme, Victoria, British Columbia.

18   For a list of emoticons, see http://enternet.com.au/techno/emoticons.html

19   For further details, see http://msc.phc.ucl.ac.uk

20   From audiotape course materials for Open University MSc in Open and Distance Education, 1999.

21   Jonassen D and Davidson M (1995) Constructivism and computer-mediated communication in distance education. *Am J Dist Educ.* **9**: 7–25.

22   Cryer P and Elton L (1998) *Conducting Small-Scale Research into Teaching and Learning in Higher Education. Resource Material for Module A.* Course text for Postgraduate Diploma in Higher Education Research and Development. University College London, London.

Part 4

Small group work in organisational settings

14

Group problem solving and decision making

> 'What is this', said the Leopard, 'that is so 'scusively dark, and yet so full of little pieces of light?'
> Rudyard Kipling, *How The Leopard Got His Spots*

Nobody's perfect

The four authors who contributed to this book have many individual deficiencies and weaknesses. One of us has no experience of management. One has creative ideas but tends to miss deadlines. Three of us can't draw. For all of these reasons, we worked as a group to solve the problem of writing this book.

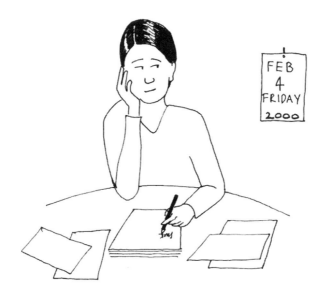

▼
One has creative ideas but tends to miss deadlines.

Until fairly recently, successful management was defined in terms of 'finding the right person for the job' and/or 'training the individual to do the job'. Organisations were preoccupied with the qualifications, experience and achievement of their individual members. Yet everyday experience tells us that the ideal individual for a given job often cannot be found – not just because they do not exist, but because they *cannot* exist. In particular, when faced with the task of solving a complex multifaceted problem, it is unlikely that any single individual will have the necessary knowledge, skills and personality to provide a truly effective solution.

Furthermore, and this is why we have included problem solving in this book, some of the qualities of a good problem solver are mutually exclusive. For example, the 'ideal problem solver' must be highly creative yet avoid becoming distracted from the task. They must be intelligent but dogged, forceful but sensitive, dynamic but patient, knowledgeable but naïve, decisive but reflective, and so on. No individual is composed entirely of strong points, and furthermore an asset that serves as a strong point in one situation can be an Achilles' heel in others. By working effectively in a team, members can contribute their individual strengths as and when they are needed. Moreover, the whole team is unlikely to step under a bus simultaneously!

A team (i.e. a group in which there is an explicit division of labour, *see* p. 4) is therefore in many ways ideally suited to problem solving. However, as illustrated in Box 14.1, Chapter 8 (*see* p. 137) and Chapter 10 (*see* p. 169), the group should not be thought of as a 'magic box'. To avoid the pitfalls described in Chapter 10 and the remainder of this chapter, the group requires clarity of purpose, an appropriate decision-making process and effective leadership. In this chapter we shall explore different types of problems, de-scribe a range of group problem-solving techniques and look at the different ways of reaching a group decision. The important issue of leadership is addressed in Chapter 17 (*see* p. 271).

Using groups in problem solving

The case study in Box 14.2 (*see* p. 228) alludes to a number of potential fault-lines in the problem-solving process. To solve a problem successfully within a group, most usually via a meeting or series of meetings, the following four factors need to be addressed.

The task

The members of the group need to understand the problem and have the expertise to solve it. They should also feel motivated and empowered to address this task, and the task itself should be one that is appropriate for group work (*see* Chapter 2, p. 28).

Group behaviour

The appropriate task and maintenance behaviours for effective group work in general should be applied. These are listed in detail in Tables 8.3 and 8.4 in Chapter 8, and they include the following:

*   gathering information
*   seeking clarification
*   proposing
*   summarising.

The decision-making method

Different methods of decision making are discussed on p. 238. There is no 'right' method, but there are certainly times when one or other of the approaches discussed below might be particularly appropriate.

The problem-solving sequence

For a problem-solving meeting to be effective, there must be an explicit structure that is adhered to by all, consisting of the following stages.

1   Define the problem.
2   Ensure that all of the relevant information has been gathered.
3   Using an appropriate decision-making approach, discuss the alternative options.
4   Choose the best option.
5   Devise an action plan.
6   Evaluate and report back.

'Tame' and 'wicked' problems

Much of the way in which we are taught to solve problems is based on rational assumptions. We take it as given that issues are capable of being dismantled, analysed and reassembled in some 'right' way. It is, after all, human nature to attempt to regulate, control or explain in some rational way anything that seems random or haphazard. The drawback of treating problems in this way is that we are at best uncomfortable (and at worst ineffectual) when handling those problems that are incapable of being reduced.

In relation to strategic planning, Horst Rittel and Melvin Webber have described the notion of 'tame' and 'wicked' problems.[1] They suggest that there are some problems which are amenable to rational description and analysis, and others that remain wicked – that is, only capable of resolution through hunch, experience and living with uncertainty.

Tame problems have most or all of the following characteristics.

- Goals are clearly defined.
- Stakeholders are identifiable.
- The values of stakeholders are accessible.
- Decision making is value driven; there are shared values among at least some stakeholders.
- Resolution depends on the collection of data and interpretation of linear information.
- The scope and outcome may be determined by modelling.
- The problem remains relatively static over time.
- The solution may be identified away from the problem (e.g. in a laboratory).
- There is a 'right' answer.

Box 14.1: Example of a tame problem – purchasing a new computer for a small department

Analyse what is happening now
Our existing PC is not able to run the latest version of statistical software. This is preventing us from analysing our research, and is generating a dependency on the IT department

Determine the required outcome
We need a PC with a Pentium III 400 MHz processor with 64 MB of RAM, and this must be within our budget of £800

Gather information
Identify possible suppliers and gather information on the various costs of their products

Identify the options
Select a number of PCs that will suit our specification

Evaluate the options
Compare the costs of these computers, taking into account their reputation for reliability and the after-sales service offered

Select one option
Choose the supplier and model that best fit our requirements

Implement the course of action
Purchase the machine

continued opposite

Evaluate the outcome
Monitor the performance and reliability of the machine

Modify action if necessary to meet requisite outcome
Deal with any adverse outcomes – for example, return a poorly functioning machine to the manufacturer

Wicked problems, in contrast, have most or all of the following characteristics.

- Some stakeholders may be unidentifiable.
- Values differ between stakeholders and over time.
- Decision making is elusive as courses open and close, and stakeholders are constantly changing.
- Information is complex and difficult to evaluate.
- Some things are unknowable.
- Outcomes are uncertain.
- The problem changes throughout the process of solution finding; the situation is likely to be volatile.
- The solution is found by action, often close to where the problem exists.
- There is no right answer – at most there is a 'best' answer.

A typical tame problem is how to cross a river. Questions like 'How many times do I need to cross it?', 'What resources do I have?' and 'Can I swim?' will determine the options for solving the problem and enable a proper decision to be made. Depending on the size of the river, the frequency of crossing and the available resources, the answers could be to swim, to build or buy a boat, to build a bridge, and so on. While the options are being analysed, the problem conveniently stays where it is until the right answer emerges.

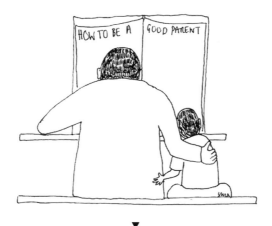

▼
Bringing up children is a typically wicked problem.

Consider, on the other hand, the 'problem' of bringing up a child. Goals will probably differ between parents, decision making occurs against a shifting background, information is lacking (but advice is not), and the only outcome that can be guaranteed is that the outcome cannot be guaranteed. The problem is changing all the time and there is no second chance to try a different approach. Bringing up a child is a typically wicked problem.

The description of some types of problem as wicked is not opting out. It identifies that a different approach is needed, as will be described in the next section.

Box 14.2: Intuitive approach to solving a wicked problem – a family with complex health and social care needs

An inner-city general practitioner takes a new family on to his list. They are refugees from a war-torn African country. The four children aged from 1 to 7 years appear malnourished, and one of them may have severe learning difficulties. The mother is pregnant, has multiple bruises, and seems to be under severe mental stress. There is no interpreter available. The GP visits the flat where they are staying and finds it squalid and overcrowded. There is an elderly relative in one of the beds, whom the family indicates does not wish to register with the practice.

Next day, the father attends the surgery, drunk and violent, apparently seeking drugs. The GP tries to involve an advocacy agency but can only get an answering machine. A commercial interpreter is found who accompanies the GP to the flat, but the GP suspects that the quality of translation is poor. The health visitor refuses to become involved until the children are tested for HIV. A social worker informs the GP that the flat is 'said to be uninhabitable' because of an allegedly unsafe gas supply. The housing officer in the council department is away on holiday.

This problem has no easy or right solution. A good start would be to pull together a multidisciplinary group, preferably including the GP, a social worker specialising in refugees and rehousing, and a professional linkworker with relevant cross-cultural knowledge. Their approach might be as follows.

Identify a range of acceptable future states
The best achievable future state is probably one in which the family is safely housed, the father is mentally stable, not engaged in criminal activity and not addicted to drugs, the children are in school, the next child is born healthy, and the mother is supported by a named keyworker who speaks her language.

Take action to generate data
The family's medical, social and economic problems need to be defined more carefully. This requires co-ordinated action by the police, the GP, the commercial interpreting agency and the social work department in the first instance.

continued opposite

Convert to information and evaluate

Once baseline medical and social data have been gathered, the different problems can be prioritised and options appraised. For example, the mother is found to be 24 weeks pregnant, anaemic and HIV-positive. The father is formally diagnosed as suffering from methadone addiction and post-traumatic stress disorder. The elderly relative is an illegal immigrant. The flat is indeed uninhabitable.

Plan within acceptable future state

An interim plan of action is constructed that includes emergency temporary rehousing, antenatal assessment and medical care for the mother, and an urgent psychiatric assessment of the father. In the longer term, there needs to be a plan for definitive housing and community support, a full medical assessment of all of the family members, educational provision for the children, and a care plan for the bed-bound elderly relative. All of these plans will need to be shaped by additional information as it accumulates. The group agree to meet again in two weeks' time.

Take next action

The family is successfully housed in temporary (bed-and-breakfast) accommodation. Antenatal care is offered and accepted. The father is registered as an addict and provided with regular methadone. He is offered psychiatric help but is reluctant to engage with it.

Generate more data

At a review meeting it is found that the bed-and-breakfast arrangement is proving difficult. Following a visit from a voluntary sector advocate several months after the referral, the father is considering joining a programme of group therapy with other refugees in his community. The mother has failed to attend for blood tests or hospital clinic appointments, apparently because of difficulties with public transport and inability to read a map. The children have not been brought for their routine immunisations and the elderly relative has disappeared.

Learn

Cultural and practical aspects of the family's complex problems were overlooked. Voluntary sector advocates, whilst committed, are often overwhelmed and may take time to deliver. All key professionals should be copied into all correspondence. A problem like this has no fairy-tale ending.

Rational vs. instinctive approaches to problem solving

The two categories of problem described above require two distinctive problem-solving approaches. Tame problems lend themselves to a rational, step-by-step process. However, wicked problems are so complex or volatile that they require action to be taken before information is generated. They need a more intuitive approach, supported by careful monitoring to determine whether progress is being made. If no progress is made, a change of approach may be needed.

The rational, step-by-step approach to problem solving generally follows this format below.

- Analyse what is happening now.
- Determine the required outcome.
- Gather information.
- Identify the options.
- Evaluate the options.
- Select one option.
- Implement the course of action.
- Evaluate the outcome.
- Modify action if necessary to meet the requisite outcome.

Where a tame problem is extensive, it may be broken down into components, each one being handled separately using the above step-by-step approach, as shown in Box 14.1.

The method for solving wicked problems requires a more instinctive approach. Consider, for example, the (hypothetical) wicked problem of finding yourself alone and lost after a stroll in the countryside has gone wrong. It is night-time, cold, very misty and sleeting heavily, and it is boggy underfoot. If you stay put you will die of hypothermia. Your objective is to reach shelter and find your way home. The staged process could involve the following steps.

- Identify a range of acceptable future states (Where do I want to be?).
- Take action to generate data (Start walking and see where I get to).
- Convert to information and evaluate (Am I any nearer to shelter and safety?).
- Plan within acceptable future state (Do I appear to be making progress? If so, carry on in the same direction; if not, change direction).
- Take next action (Walk some distance further).
- Generate more data (Where am I now?).
- Learn (What things have helped me and what things have hindered me?).

This intuitive approach to solving wicked problems is illustrated in Box 14.2 using a case history.

Many heads better than one?

There is a rapidly developing literature that describes the potential increase in productivity that can occur in the work environment when individuals share goals and work in teams.[2–5] However, whilst group work *can* improve productivity and aid the decision-making process, there is substantial evidence that the output of the group can sometimes be worse than the output of the most competent individual within the group, and even occasionally worse than the *average* performance of the individual members. There are also plenty of examples of group decisions that are fundamentally flawed to the point of being potentially dangerous (*see* the examples in Chapter 10, p. 166, including an account of how the Bay of Pigs and Challenger disasters may have been caused by poor group processes).[6] Box 14.3 summarises some key evidence from experimental psychology in this field.

Box 14.3:   Evidence from problem-solving experiments in the laboratory

There is a vast literature from experimental psychology on what happens when individuals and groups are given problems to solve in the laboratory. The relevance of these experimental studies to real-life problem solving is hotly debated.

In experimental problem-solving situations, groups perform better than their average member in numerical estimation-type tasks – indeed, they generally perform to the level of the best individual member, since that person generates a solution which the others recognise as correct (i.e. a 'eureka'-type situation).[7] In problems that involve puzzles or brainteasers, group performance is better than that of the average individual member, but worse than that of the best member. In more complex laboratory-based tasks, groups frequently exceed the performance of the 'average judgement' and at times surpass the performance of the best member. One key determinant of above average performance by the group is the extent to which the group has worked together on a task that is important to all of the members.[8]

Apart from the nature of the task itself, the two most significant contributors to poor group decisions in experimental situations are inadequate sharing of information and inappropriate group norms. It has been found that groups concentrate on the information that is shared at an early stage of a problem evaluation, and that individual members do not generally share all of the information that they have at the outset. Because of this, important data is often left unconsidered, and the group may lull itself into a false sense of security and competence – a situation which Janis termed 'groupthink' (*see* Chapter 10, p. 166).

As a general observation, groups make riskier decisions in laboratory conditions than individuals – a phenomenon known as the 'risky shift' process. This tendency for groups to take more extreme positions than individuals has

continued overleaf

resulted in work on 'polarisation' and 'depolarisation' within groups and how these processes occur. Most people favour the theory of 'persuasive arguments' to explain this trend. Positions or solutions that at first seem favourable are taken up by successive group members, and more and better arguments are put forward for the favoured position than for any other possible outcome. This effect increases with the novelty and perceived validity of the arguments put forward. The effect is maximal when there are more members for than members against the proposed solution, and the theory is further strengthened by the fact that 'depolarisation' (a shift towards moderation or compromise) occurs when two equal-sized factions within groups disagree. It has also been found that many factors influence this process.

Summarising the experimental research in this area, Levine notes that normative processes (the adjustments that group members make in order to achieve social desirability) are more likely when a practical judgement needs to be made, an explicit aim of the group is to achieve harmony, and there is a need for a public (external) response to a problem. In contrast, the influence of information, its availability and quality will be more likely when the task itself is an intellectual one, the group puts greater emphasis on addressing the task than on achieving harmony, and the group works in a private forum.[9]

Although any conclusions drawn from experimental work must be tentative, it surely follows from the above evidence that groups which seek to make decisions and/or solve complex problems must be aware of the *process* as well as the *content* of their deliberations, and employ a more sophisticated mechanism for sharing information, voicing and managing dissent and reaching conclusions than simple discussion. If you are interested in this field of research, we recommend two sources which summarise how the conditions under which experimental groups operate may influence the way in which members contribute and modify their views, how alliances form, how minorities and majorities shape the group norms, and how information is shared.[10,11]

Problem-solving techniques

When a problem is complex, and especially when different members of the group have different perspectives on it, a solution may well not emerge spontaneously, even with good behaviour and skilled facilitation within the group. We shall now describe three techniques for analysing complex problems, namely force field analysis, fishbone diagrams and future basing.

Force field analysis

Force field analysis is credited to Kurt Lewin.[12] The technique was developed to aid problem diagnosis where the problem is regarded as dynamic and the present situation capable of being changed. The model assumes that there is a present state, or equilibrium, and it catalogues the forces for and against change (*see* Figure 14.1).

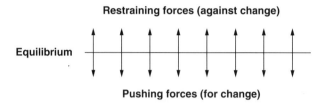

Figure 14.1:   Force field analysis.

The steps involved in carrying out a force field analysis are as follows.

1   Identify the problem and write it down.
2   Define the problem in specific terms (Who is involved? How big is it?).
3   Describe what outcome is ideally required.
4   List the forces pushing for change.
5   List the restraining forces.
6   In the following order, consider how to:
    • reduce restraining forces
    • identify new pushing forces
    • identify which new pushing forces will encounter least resistance
    • divert restraining forces to other issues
    • identify any pushing forces which may have created the problem in the first place by ensuring resistance.

A strategy for change should now be clearer, based on where to enable the withdrawal of a restraining force, where to apply pressure and where to withdraw pressure. The strategy should also include time-scales and the resources needed to achieve the goal. As a general rule, there is far more to be gained from identifying and reducing the restraining forces than from increasing the pushing forces. For an excellent example of the use of force field analysis in introducing new ways of learning in higher education, see Elton's recent paper.[13]

Fishbone diagrams

The fishbone diagram, also known as the cause-and-effect diagram, is probably the commonest method of analysing problems used by problem-solving groups. It is a means of separating causes from effects, and is of great assistance to groups in viewing a problem in its totality. When completed, it resembles the skeleton of a fish. Many problems take on a different perspective when viewed in this way. Causes which previously appeared to be central often fade in importance as the group's analysis brings the key causes to light. Figure 14.2 shows a fishbone diagram from a paper on total quality management in healthcare by Berwick, Bunker and Enthoven.[14] It examines the problem of late transfer of data from the emergency room to the medical office in an American hospital.

There are six steps involved in the construction of the fishbone diagram.

Step 1: Draw the head (the effect)

Write the effect on the right-hand side of a large sheet of paper. Make sure that the effect chosen is as clear and precise as possible. The more general the effect, the more general the causes will be, and this often makes it difficult to get the group to engage with the problem. Problem-solving groups are concerned with actually getting things done rather than talking about them in vague and general terms, so they do need to get down to identifying the detailed causes of the problem.

Step 2: Draw the ribs (up to eight suggested causes)

Draw the main ribs of the fish, and write in the headings of the main problem areas. Experience shows that around six to eight headings are adequate for the majority of situations encountered. In the example shown in Figure 14.2, these are determined by following the 'flow' of information through the system – identifying, labelling, copying, sorting, transfer and arrival.

Step 3: Set the scene for creative activity

The group should remind itself of the rules of brainstorming and write them up somewhere so that everyone can see them.

Step 4: Brainstorm

Use the rules and procedures of brainstorming to generate a list of the things that can go wrong at each stage. These should be written down along the 'ribs' of the fish skeleton. The person doing the writing needs to concentrate on putting the ideas on the diagram under the right headings. Group members should take responsibility for ensuring that their own suggestions and those of other members are recorded on the diagram.

Step 5: Incubate

Allow the ideas on the diagram to incubate for a while, to enable them to sink in and ensure that none of the suggestions are rejected out of hand. This can

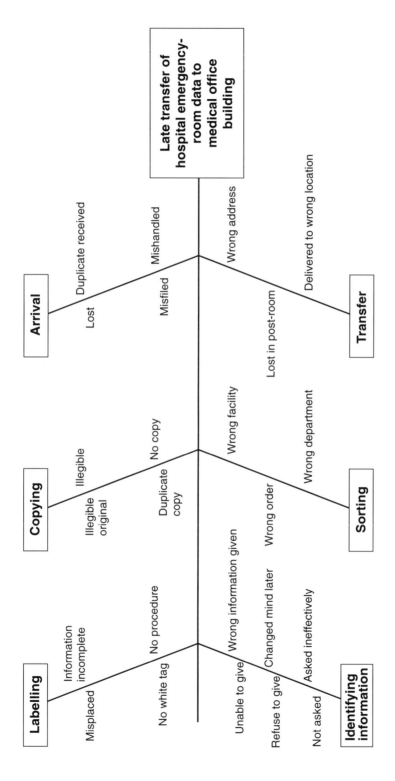

Figure 14.2: Fishbone diagram to analyse late data transfer in a hospital.[14]

be done by sitting quietly for ten minutes thinking about the implications of the completed diagram. Alternatively, put the sheet in a clearly visible location in the workplace between group meetings and think about it during the week. Of the two options, the second is preferable, not only because it gives more time to incubate, but also because it gives other people in the organisation who are not group members a valuable chance to see the output and to contribute to it if they wish to do so.

Step 6: Analyse

The next stage is to analyse the whole diagram. Here the group should look at the analysis and decide which ideas and groups of ideas 'jump off the page'. The Pareto principle (an established tenet of management theory initially proposed by an Italian economist[15]) states that about 20% of the causes are likely to account for 80% of the effect, and it is these few causes that the group is looking for at this stage. At this point, the group has not collected data and is using its knowledge and experience to determine the essential areas on which to focus with regard to data collection.

For example, if we believe that the main cause of the late transfer is incorrect labelling, illegible writing and poor copying, we must then design a protocol (and training) for key staff in the emergency room to ensure that labelling will be improved.

Future basing

The traditional way to solve a problem is to start where you are and work forwards from there – that is, to define the present problem, analyse it and work forward in a step-wise way (*see* Figure 14.3). Future basing is a technique that encourages the group to imagine an ideal future scenario (i.e. one in which the problem is not present), describe that future, and plan actions to bring that situation about (*see* Figure 14.4).[16]

Conclusion

Group work is not a panacea for decision making or problem solving. The skilled use of the group process can make the output of a group greater than the sum of the contributions of individual members. However, a poorly run group makes poor decisions and solves few problems. In particular, discussion and dissent within a group can be managed productively using formal techniques for promoting creativity (brainstorming), developing consensus (guided

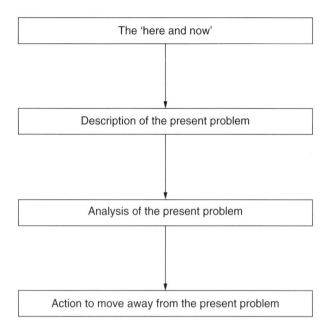

Figure 14.3: Traditional problem-solving sequence.

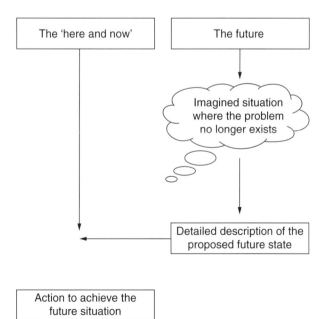

Figure 14.4: Future-based problem-solving sequence.

discussion and nominal group process), systematically appraising assumptions and recommendations (dialectical inquiry and devil's advocacy) and representing complex problems (force field analysis, fishbone diagrams and future basing).

The decision-making process

Sandberg and colleagues have outlined three well-known methods for reducing the tendency towards normative trends and lack of information exchange that typify poor decisions.[17] These are:

* consensus processes
* dialectical inquiry
* devil's advocacy.

These methods are summarised below. We suggest that additional techniques described in Chapter 5, such as crossover groups (*see* p. 80), brainstorming (*see* p. 91) and reverse brainstorming (*see* p. 92) can also help to maximise the creativity and output of the group.

Consensus processes

Guided discussion

This unstructured method allows every member to participate in a free exchange of ideas and opinions, followed by explanations, discussion and agreement. This method calls for high levels of communication skill, and requires group members to recognise the merit of other people's ideas, avoid posing win–lose situations, be flexible, and avoid being fooled by initial agreements. The following guidelines are used.

* Each individual should have an opportunity to present their ideas to the group.
* Assumptions and data underlying opinions should be explored – not just the opinions themselves.
* Discussion should be open and constructive.

Nominal group technique

This structured decision-making method involves a staged generation, clarification and comparison, and sequential votes on ideas and suggestions. It is discussed in detail in relation to research in Chapter 19 (*see* pp. 305–8).

Dialectic inquiry

This method is essentially a structured method of discussing pros and cons. The group is divided into two equal-sized subgroups, each of which develops one side of the argument and presents the relevant assumptions and recommendations. In this way, the group should be able to separate out the underlying operating principles. The key steps are as follows.

- One group (subgroup 1) is asked to develop their assumptions and recommendations as rapidly as possible (within 15 minutes or so). The second group awaits their decisions.
- Subgroup 1 presents its assumptions and recommendations to subgroup 2, and provides them with a written list. Subgroup 1 describes the supporting arguments for their case.
- The subgroups separate and move to different physical spaces in order to develop an opposing alternative. Subgroup 2 should develop a reasoned set of opposing recommendations and opposing arguments. Again the assumptions should be clarified and they should be different to the assumptions underpinning the recommendations of subgroup 1.
- Subgroup 2 presents its assumptions and recommendations to subgroup 1, and provides a copy of their recommendations.
- The subgroups then debate the two alternatives. At this point, the assumptions should be exposed again and explored. Through group discussion, agreement is sought on the final list of assumptions, which will include items from the original lists, revisions, and new assumptions that have surfaced during the debate.
- Using this final list of assumptions, the entire group should develop a set of recommendations. This may involve considerable debate. It is important not to record the resulting recommendations until there is agreement that it is appropriate to close the discussions.

Devil's advocacy

The group is again divided into two equal-sized subgroups, but this time one group systematically probes and critiques each element of the assumptions, arguments and recommendations that are put forward by the other group. The key steps are as follows.

- Assign members to the 'recommendations' and 'devil's advocate' subgroups and arrange different physical spaces in which they can work.
- The 'recommendations' subgroup produces a reasoned set of recommendations and arguments. Their assumptions should be clarified and listed.

- The 'devil's advocate' subgroup independently discusses the case or problem and explores the arguments and weaknesses they can foresee.
- The two groups come together. The 'recommendations' subgroup makes a brief presentation and provides a list of their recommendations and supporting arguments.
- The groups separate again and the 'devil's advocate' subgroup develops a logical, plausible critique of the other subgroup's recommendations. They should try to identify problems with the assumptions and information that underlie the 'recommendations' subgroup's decisions. This process should take no more than approximately 15 or 20 minutes.
- The two subgroups come together again. The 'devil's advocate' subgroup provides a copy of its critique and explains the main points briefly.
- The two subgroups stay together and work towards an agreement. The 'recommendations' subgroup revises its plans in the light of valid arguments. Again these revisions are open to reasoned critiques and the revision/critique/revision cycles should continue until both subgroups agree to a final set of recommendations.

Acceptance of group decisions

Whatever the decision-making process, it is crucially important to feed back formally to the group the outcome of their decision-making meeting. It may well be found that, although a solution was 'agreed' on, it has failed to be successful (e.g. because the group decision was not actually accepted by individuals who chose to remain silent). If there is not a total consensus on the decision, it will be more difficult to implement it.

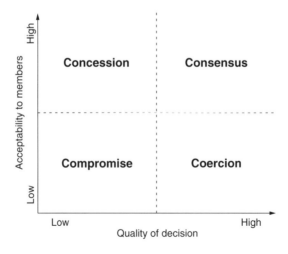

Figure 14.5: Types of group decisions.

The levels of acceptance of group decisions are illustrated in Figure 14.5. They can be broadly divided into the following four categories:

- *compromise* – 'Lowest common denominator'; offends no one, commits no one and is unlikely to result in commitment to action
- *coercion* – pressure on weaker members to bend to the task; high-quality decision but uneven commitment to action
- *concession* – acceptance of the need to agree in order to obtain commitment to action, but the decision may bear little relation to the task in hand
- *consensus* – subject matter is talked through with a clear grasp of the task in hand. Exploration continues until there is an even commitment to an appropriate course of action.

Conclusion

As we suggested in Chapter 1 (*see* p. 16), many heads can often be better than one for addressing a problem or reaching a difficult decision. However, a valid solution or a high-quality decision cannot be produced simply by throwing the problem at the group and asking them to 'fight it out'. Attention to the group process (*see* Chapter 8, p. 137) is of the utmost importance, skilled facilitation is often needed, and formal problem-solving and decision-making techniques should be employed, especially if the group is addressing an issue that fulfils the criteria for a 'wicked problem' (*see* p. 225).

References

1   Rittel HWJ and Webber MM (1969) Dilemmas in a general theory of planning. *Policy Sci.* **4**: 155–73.

2   Belbin RM (1981) *Management Teams*. Butterworth Heinemann, Oxford.

3   Dyer WG (1994) *Team Building*. Addison-Wesley, Reading, MA.

4   West M (1994) *Effective Teamwork*. British Psychological Society, Leicester.

5   Robbins H and Finley M (1995) *Why Teams Don't Work*. Pacesetter Books, Princeton, NJ.

6   Hill GW (1982) Group versus individual performance: are *N* + 1 heads better than one? *Psychol Bull.* **91**: 517–39.

7   Hastie R (1986) Review essay: experimental evidence on group accuracy. In: G Owen and B Grofman (eds) *Information Pooling and Group Decision Making*. JAI Press, Westport, CT.

8 Watson WE, Michaelsen LK and Sharp W (1991) Member competence, group interaction and group decision making: a longitudinal study. *J Appl Psychol.* **76**: 803–9.

9 Levine JM and Moreland RL (1998) Small groups. In: *Handbook of Social Psychology.* McGraw-Hill, Boston, MA.

10 Moscovivi S and Lage E (1976) Studies in social influence. III. Majority versus minority influence in a group. *Eur J Soc Psychol.* **6**: 149–74.

11 Strasser G, Stewart DD and Wittenbaum GM (1992) Expert roles and information exchange during discussion: the importance of knowing who knows what. *J Exp Soc Psychol.* **31**: 244–65.

12 Lewin K (1952) *Field Theory in Social Science.* Tavistock, London.

13 Elton L (1999) New ways of learning in higher education: managing the change. *Tertiary Educ Manag.* **5**: 207–25.

14 Berwick DM, Enthoven A and Bunker JP (1992) Quality management in the NHS: the doctor's role – I. *BMJ.* **304**: 235–9.

15 Turner JR (1995) *The Handbook of Project-Based Management.* McGraw-Hill, London.

16 Gorman P (1998) *Managing Multidisciplinary Teams in the NHS.* Kogan Page, London.

17 Sandberg WR, Schweiger DM and Ragan JW (1986) Group approaches for improving strategic decision making. *Acad Manag J.* **29**: 51–7.

15

Groups across boundaries: multidisciplinary and multi-agency team working

> *Then they came to lands where people spoke strangely, and sang songs*
> *that Bilbo had never heard before.*
> JRR Tolkein, *The Hobbit*

Why have multidisciplinary groups or teams?

This chapter draws heavily on three sources produced specifically with multidisciplinary teams in mind, namely Paul Gorman's *Managing Multidisciplinary Teams in the NHS*,[1] Peter and James Pritchard's *Teamwork for Primary and Shared Care*[2] and Øvretveit's works on multidisciplinary teamwork in healthcare.[3,4]

Perhaps, incidentally, it is no accident that much of the research work on multidisciplinary teams has been done in the healthcare sector. As one of us noted recently:

> *Teams in healthcare settings are often expected to muddle through, solving problems of co-ordination and differences of professional interest. Calling professionals a team has become a way in which managers and planners avoid the real problems and work needed to co-ordinate an increasingly complex range of services in the community. Forging a team out of a diverse set of professionals requires structural and managerial shifts not yet visible in current practice, and few attempts have been made to consider the structural difficulties in health planning or policy reviews.*[5]

Multidisciplinarity is more than political correctness, and in today's world it cannot be avoided. Within our organisations we are often required to manage teams or chair committees across professional, disciplinary and departmental boundaries. Those in senior and middle management (and that means most people who might read this book) are increasingly required to work effectively across boundaries in order to run inter-agency projects, deal with complex problems or cases and develop better structures for collaborative working. Most of us sit on at least one committee or working group whose members are drawn from a range of different professional backgrounds and/or different departments and organisations. We can probably all recall frustrating or ineffective encounters within this type of group.

Gorman describes five core benefits of working in a multidisciplinary or multi-agency team, rather than as separate individuals or groups each tackling a different part of the problem. These advantages are as follows:

- *better quality decisions in complex areas* – by using information from all relevant contributors, there is less danger of decisions being taken in ignorance of vital data
- *clear roles and responsibilities* – if everyone is together when roles and responsibilities are allocated, these are more likely to be agreed, transparent and understood
- *greater commitment to the agreed plan* – ownership of decisions is better when stakeholders have personally contributed to them
- *one team, one voice* – all team members will hopefully be 'singing from the same hymn-sheet'
- *mutual support and encouragement* – working relationships should become co-operative rather than competitive, and there will be a team identity and team spirit.

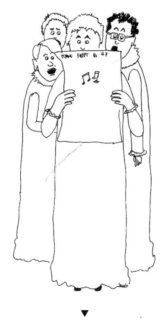

▼

Singing from the same hymn sheet.

Pritchard and Pritchard, writing specifically about multidisciplinary teams involved in the care of patients, add five additional points, some of which clearly have relevance beyond the healthcare field:

- *skill mix* – rare skills are used more appropriately
- *continuity* – care delivered by a team ensures greater continuity than that delivered by an individual
- *standards* – peer influence and informal leading raise the standards of care
- *fulfilment* – team members have more job satisfaction and cope better with failure
- *holistic care* – team-working allows co-ordination of preventive work with caring and curing activities.

Special challenges of multidisciplinary teams

No one should make the mistake of assuming that running a multidisciplinary, interdepartmental or inter-agency team will be easy. However, by addressing and overcoming barriers that arise *within* the team, members may create the potential to transcend barriers that exist *beyond* the team between their different disciplines, departments or organisations.

Gorman suggests three dimensions of effectiveness in multidisciplinary teams (*see* Figure 15.1), namely structural, cultural and interpersonal.

The structural dimension includes formal organisational issues. What status, level of autonomy, rewards, physical and practical constraints and

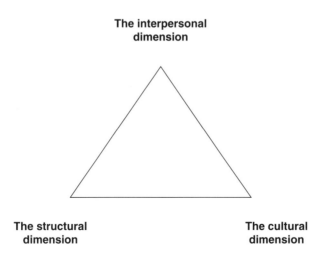

Figure 15.1: Gorman's three dimensions of multidisciplinary working.

lines of accountability do different team members have within their separate professions or organisations? Where does each team member sit in his or her own organisational or professional hierarchy? And where does their organisation or profession sit in the wider hierarchy?

The cultural dimension encompasses much of what we have described as the 'baggage' which people (often unconsciously) bring to a group or team (*see* p. 23). What are their professional (or commercial) ideologies, allegiances, rationales, value systems and expectations? What aspects of the problem are they likely to view as important, and what are they likely to dismiss as irrelevant or incomprehensible? This is discussed further below.

The interpersonal dimension – whether two or more individuals 'get on' with one another – may be easy to spot but difficult to define or change. In many cases, differences are perceived as interpersonal when in reality they arise from structural or cultural dimensions. For example, a senior man in a team may come across as aloof and patronising (and perhaps even sexist) when he asks a more junior female colleague to contact him via his secretary, but this request might be interpreted differently if all of the team members had their own secretary.

Group, team, network or collaboration?

We mentioned in Chapter 1 (*see* p. 4) that the terms 'group' and 'team' are frequently used interchangeably, but that we ourselves feel that teams are characterised by explicit role differentiation. As Table 15.1 shows, teams

Table 15.1: Comparison of different aspects of groups, teams, collaborations, committees and task forces

	Group	*Team*	*Network*	*Collaboration*	*Committee*	*Task force*
Relative size	+	+ (variable)	+++	+++	++	+
Boundaries (e.g. closed membership)	+++	+++	+	++	++++	+++
Hierarchical?	+	++	+	++	++++	+++
Shared identity	++++	++++	+	++	+++	++++
Role differentiation	++	++++	+	+	+++	+++
Task orientation	++	++++	+	+	++	++++
Cohesion	+++	+++	+	++	+	++++
Orientation to external agencies	+	++	+	++	++++	+++
Social orientation	+++	++	++++	+	+	++
Interaction between members	++++	++++	++	+	+	+++
Time limited?	++	+++	+	+	+	++++

+ ⟷ ++++ = level of characteristic specified
Low   High

are also perhaps more task-oriented than groups. Other common multidisciplinary groupings include committees (very formal with strict membership criteria), task forces (as the name suggests, highly task-oriented) and collaborations (more dynamic and potentially flexible interactions between individuals or organisations). Not all of these 'groupings' merit the title 'group', as it is often very apparent that the members of a committee or board do not share perspectives or agree on objectives!

Øvretveit has developed a complex taxonomy of teams and similar groupings in the work setting. These include the following.[4]

- *Network-association teams* – these are informal and (usually) voluntary groupings in which people who have a common interest in a problem get together to solve it. They may already know each other, although probably not intimately (social networks are characterised by distant rather than close links between members).[6] One example is the various subdivisions of the Human Genome Project – an international academic and scientific network of individuals working to decode the human genome. The members of the different subgroups all know (or *know of*) one another via their publications and presentations at meetings, and many of them have friendships dating back to their university days. Communication across different parts of this network when a particular subject query arises is generally rapid and effective, and is based on both personal and professional ties. Network-association teams rarely have a nominated leader, and their members are generally not 'line-managed' by another network member.
- *Formal multidisciplinary teams* – these are fully managed and official groupings with agreed membership, governed by an agreed and explicit team policy that is upheld by a designated team leader. This structure can often be found in psychiatric hospitals, in which each patient has a care team including a psychiatrist, psychiatric nurse, art therapist, social worker, and so on. The team holds regular meetings to share reports and plan patient care.
- *Complex teams* – in some teams, not all of the members share the same relationship with the leader. For example, Øvretveit describes the 'managed core and co-ordinated associate team' in which the core team members are directly managed by the leader, but which includes several additional members who act as associates. The best example of this is probably the typical UK primary healthcare team, which has a core staff of practice nurses, receptionists and administrators employed by and answerable to the doctors, but also includes a range of attached staff such as health visitors, district nurses, social workers and perhaps even alternative therapists.

Many multidisciplinary groupings are described as teams when they are in reality nothing of the kind. There is a temptation to use the word 'team' for groupings characterised by a much larger size and lower degree of cohesion and integration than is generally associated with the term – and hence to convey an image of teamwork where none exists! Perhaps we should be both braver and more explicit. For example, if the grouping fits the characteristics of a collaboration or a network we should make sure that we use the correct term. The 'primary healthcare team' would, in certain more extreme cases, be better described as the 'collection of loosely associated individuals who share a staff-room and/or sometimes pass by one another in the same building'!

Øvretveit echoed this sentiment:

> *Certain problems and behaviours will be encountered if the structure is wrong, regardless of who works in the structure. People come and go, but the problems will remain. Problems of structure are not overcome by calling a group a team.*[3]

Whatever its detailed structure, the successful team is characterised by clear goals (everyone knows what the team is doing), clear roles (everyone knows what they as individuals are doing), the right mix of skills and experience, mutual trust, and a belief among all members that there is something in it for them.

Communication and the multidisciplinary team

One person's specialist language is another's impenetrable jargon, and one person's humour is another's bad taste. In our experience, one of the most irritating aspects of multidisciplinary working, and a source of needless frustration and stress, is the use of language that is potentially inflammatory. This behaviour may be deliberate or inadvertent, but it will not go unnoticed. Examples we have encountered which reflect cultural differences between professions, genders and social classes include the following:

1 formality and tortuosity – for example:
    • 'I proceeded to the paediatric ward and ascertained that the minor was in bed, whereupon I commenced my interrogation' (police-officer)
    • 'We need to downsize this organisation' (middle manager)
2 referring to things by an official name or number when they could easily be described in lay language – for example:
    • 'He came to see me for a Med 3 [sick note] and an FP10 [prescription]' (doctor)
    • 'I could upload the compressed graphic file [I could put that picture on the website]' (computer technician)

3   excessive use of acronyms – for example:
   - 'The patient was admitted with a BBA [born before arrival]' (midwife)
   - 'What we need for the summative assessment is MCQs rather than MEQs' (educationalist)
4   sexist, racist, ageist or other potentially exclusive language – for example:
   - 'I've recently got a new car and she's just so smooth' (sales representative)
   - 'You're really going to have to work like a black to meet that deadline' (company chairman)
5   naïve stereotyping – for example:
   - 'He was a nasty, incompetent little man – probably a left-wing homosexual' (headmaster)
6   manipulation of language to make a political or ideological point – for example:
   - 'I read it in the *New Statesperson*' (feminist)
   - 'Does anyone else want a dead animal sandwich before I throw them away?' (vegetarian)
7   use of emotive symbols or metaphors – for example:
   - 'Suppose this plate is me and Fred, then you're the mustard pot' (team leader to somewhat prickly junior colleague)
   - 'we've got to show them that our willy is bigger than theirs' (young male negotiator explaining strategy to three female staff).

If you are facilitating or chairing a multidisciplinary team, one important aspect of your role is to anticipate difficulties in communication and, perhaps by playing the ignorant fool, ask a speaker to clarify or modify their point. You may wish to invite the team to draw up some ground rules on this topic (*see* p. 102) at the outset, and you should also, if necessary, approach individuals outside the group and suggest (with examples) how they could modify their use of language and metaphor.

'Professional' vs. 'management' cultures

The words we use are just one example of 'how we do things in our profession (or other group)'. Consider, for example, teenage culture. It includes not just a set of 'in' expressions, but also hairstyles, clothes, jewellery, music, food and a whole set of values and expectations about the world.

   Professional culture is somewhat different, but is equally encompassing. Professionals dress in a certain way, read particular newspapers, and use a very characteristic body language (of which they are usually unconscious). Furthermore, as Box 15.1 shows, they take pride in what they define as their standards, and they undertake as a profession to police those standards. They assume certain ethical and moral principles to be self-evident, and have

---

Box 15.1:   Features of professionals (adapted from Simon)[7]

Professionals possess a body of knowledge and skills based on long periods of training. These skills and knowledge are demanded by society. Professionals also share a code of ethics that indicates how patients and clients should be served and the social attitudes that should be accepted.

Six key features define a professional.

1   There is a body of knowledge or skill held as a common possession and united by extended effort.
2   There is an educational process based on this body of knowledge for which the professional group as a whole has a recognised responsibility.
3   There is a standard of qualification for admission to the professional group based on character, training and proved competence.
4   There is a standard of conduct with regard to courtesy, honour and ethics which guides the practitioner in his or her relationships with clients, colleagues and the public.
5   There is a more-or-less formal recognition of status by colleagues and by the state as a basis of good standing.
6   The organisation of the professional group should be devoted to its common advancement and its social duty, rather than to the maintenance of an economic policy.

---

difficulty in comprehending people who feel differently. As the previous section illustrated, they also develop and become trapped within their own professional language, humour and social conventions. Management culture is fundamentally quite different, as shown in Table 15.2, and trade-union culture is different again (*see* Chapter 8, p. 140).

Table 15.2:   Differences between professionals and managers (adapted from Simon)[7]

	Professionals	*Managers*
Expertise	Narrow	Broad
	Specific to a particular topic or subtopic	Specific to a particular organisation
	Transferable across organisations	Transferable within the organisation
Status	Often an independent contractor	Usually an employee
Allegiance	To own profession	To own organisation
Skills and training	Defined, co-ordinated and assessed by own profession	Defined, co-ordinated and assessed by the organisation
Career advancement	Generally via external labour market (beyond the organisation)	Often via internal labour market (within the organisation)
Discipline/ enforcement of standards	By professional body	By line manager within the organisation
Values	Oriented towards the profession's perceived social duty	Oriented towards the (economic) advancement of the organisation

For example, the nurses, managers and doctors on a multidisciplinary healthcare team may be entirely unaware that they are displaying behaviour patterns and making assumptions that the other subgroups do not share. This can lead to niggling problems in small and apparently unimportant aspects of group work. For instance, the nurses may be quite comfortable each bringing their own packed lunch to a meeting, while the managers might assume that everyone will go to the canteen, and some of the consultants might expect to go out to a restaurant. Small clashes like this lead at first to surprise, then to an unconscious feeling that 'I don't like working like this' and then, as the small irritations accumulate, to suppressed resentment. Most often in the health service, culture clashes occur between clinicians (doctors, nurses and others who work with patients) and managers.

It should not be assumed that professional culture is a bad thing, or that all members of the team must be stripped of their 'baggage' before effective team-work can begin. Such an approach (which formed the basis of the 'T-group' approach that was popular in the 1970s)[8] is impractical, unhelpful and probably damaging. The role of the facilitator is to encourage a deeper awareness of cultural 'baggage' in general, so that each member not only understands and respects where the others in the team are coming from, but also shows an awareness of where they themselves are coming from and how this stance is likely to be perceived by their colleagues. Teenage culture is easy to identify because (for most of us) it jars with our own set of assumptions and values. To become aware of one's own cultural baggage requires a special reflective technique which anthropologists call 'making the familiar strange'. It involves asking the question 'How would *others* interpret what I am saying/doing now?'.

Note, by the way, that we all belong to several different cultures (or subcultures). The 'baggage' that an individual might bring to a multidisciplinary team as a community pharmacist is different to but overlaps with the 'baggage' they have from being (say) middle class, Jewish or the mother of a young baby. In the National Health Service, where professionals often also play management roles (e.g. clinical directors), allegiances and values may conflict or blur within an individual. For this and other reasons, 'professional culture' should not be regarded as either static or deterministic, and both the facilitator and the team members must consciously avoid stereotyping.

Facilitating multidisciplinary teams

It is often said that multidisciplinary groups need a special type of facilitator. In fact, the principles of leading or facilitating this type of group are no different to those for any other type of group (*see* Chapter 4, p. 55) or any other type of problem-solving process (*see* Chapter 14, p. 224). However, in multidisciplinary teams the task is generally more challenging, and if you are not yet fully confident about your facilitation skills, we advise you to stick to unidisciplinary groups for the time being!

The theoretical steps involved in leading a multidisciplinary team in a task-related or problem-solving activity are shown in Figure 15.2. The problem is that multidisciplinary working is rarely this straightforward. The devil fools with the best-laid plans. Common difficulties include the following.

- *Members* – membership of your team probably goes with the role rather than the individual, and you may well find that the representative who joins you for the first meeting is replaced before the project is complete.
- *Attendance* – poor attendance is more common when team members are geographically distant and each member has a different set of conflicting demands on their time.
- *Conflicting loyalties* – some of the members may have been sent to join your team in order to further the agenda of their professional group or organisation. They may have no personal commitment to the task which your team has been set – indeed, they may be there primarily to try to stop the team taking a particular course of action! Even if this is not the case, there is an inevitable tension between the autonomy of the team to make a decision and the ability of the individual members to take that decision back to their own organisations and implement it.
- *Lack of resources* – almost all teams believe that they need more resources than they have at present. In multidisciplinary or trans-organisational teams, resources may have been pulled together from a variety of sources, and there may be a 'turf war' over how much should be contributed by each organisation or interest group.
- *Culture clashes* – as discussed above, members may view the world (and the task) from very different perspectives. With effective facilitation, this conflict can be used productively in the group process. You should encourage your team members to go beyond their emotional responses to cultural differences and use them as positive learning experiences. This is what multidisciplinarity is all about!
- *Managing without authority* – if you are leading a unidisciplinary, single-organisation team, the chances are that you are the boss. You may well be the direct line manager of everyone in your team. However, as the facilitator, leader or chairperson of a multidisciplinary or inter-organisational team, the only authority you have is by consensus and influence, and you must adopt a style which is appropriate to that reality.

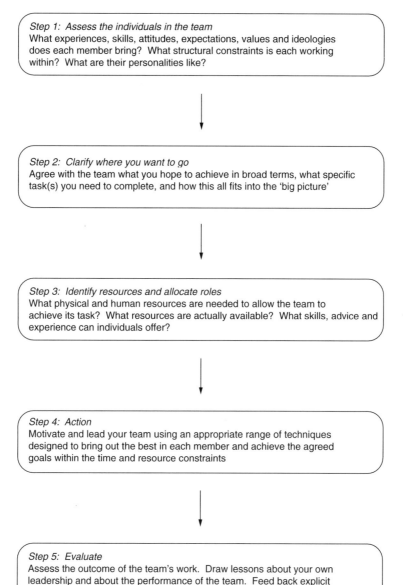

Figure 15.2:   Managing multidisciplinary teams (adapted from Gorman).[1]

Successful teamwork across organisational boundaries

There is certainly no simple blueprint for success, but Gorman notes that the following features tend to characterise successful inter-agency partnerships.

*   *Reciprocity* – there should be something in it for all of the players.
*   *A convener* – someone with credibility and who is respected within all of the agencies involved, and who understands all of the perspectives, should act as convener.
*   *Addressing all levels* – the partnership should work at all levels in the different agencies. For example, if the team involves predominantly middle management, there should also be support from senior management and a sensitivity to the perspective of the front-line staff whose job it will be to implement any agreements that are made.
*   *Managing differences* – we mentioned earlier the cultural differences between professional groups and organisations. These differences should be managed honestly, and conflicts of interest brought 'up front'.
*   *Working within structures* – too often, bureaucratic and unwieldy new structures are created for multi-agency working. If possible, the existing administrative structures should be used or adapted.
*   *Task orientation* – it is much easier to shelter behind policy documents, mission statements and other comfortable generalisations than to focus on real tasks with real deadlines. Continually looking to a future product from the team is essential for such a product to appear.

Box 15.2 suggests some ways to make a multidisciplinary interorganisational 'team' fail.

Box 15.2:   Ten ways to make a multidisciplinary team fail (adapted from Øvretveit)[3]

1   Practitioners continue to work and meet together as a single-profession group, just as they did before they were told that they would each be working in a multidisciplinary team.
2   Each profession or professional group continues to operate their own referral procedures and work priorities.
3   Professional managers maintain close control over practitioners – allocating work, recruiting team members, deciding training and reviewing cases.
4   Many of the participants are only part-time members of the team, with the rest of their time being allocated to one or more different areas or services.

continued opposite

---

5   There is no team base – contact and communication points, records and secretarial support are all at different sites.

6   There is no team leader position with a responsibility for team operations.

7   There are no team objectives or priorities, but only general statements of intent.

8   There is no decision-making procedure within the team for processes, workload management, management issues or the development of planning proposals.

9   There is no formal annual review by higher management of team operation and achievements.

10 There is no plan for wider service of which the team is a part, and no individual or group with a clear responsibility for creating such a plan. The group is drawn into work which the purchaser will not pay and which is the responsibility of other providers.

Evaluating multidisciplinary teamwork

The general principles of evaluation, described in detail in Chapter 9, apply equally to multidisciplinary and cross-boundary teams. In addition, such teams might consider the following additional aspects (or areas of emphasis) of their success, as suggested by Poulton and West:[9]

*   the views and experiences of their clients or service users
*   the innovativeness of the team
*   the extent of team vision and shared objectives
*   'participative safety' (i.e. the extent to which the team is regarded by members as supportive and that information is safe within the team)
*   commitment to excellence – a shared concern for the quality of both team and individual performance.

Pritchard and Pritchard have explored this agenda in more detail and suggest some short questionnaires with which it is possible to attempt to address these aspects of teamwork.[2] Anderson and West's 'team climate' inventory may also be worth attempting.[10]

References

1   Gorman P (1998) *Managing Multidisciplinary Teams in the NHS*. Kogan Page, London.

2   Pritchard P and Pritchard J (1994) *Teamwork for Primary and Shared Care: a Practical Workbook* (2e). Oxford Medical Publications, Oxford.

3   Øvretveit J (1986) *Organising Multidisciplinary Community Teams*. HCS Working Paper, Brunel University. BIOSS, Uxbridge.

4   Øvretveit J (1993) *Co-ordinating Community Care*. Open University Press, Milton Keynes.

5   Elwyn G, Rapport FL and Kinnersley P (1998) Re-engineering the primary health care team. *J Interprof Care*. **12**: 189–98.

6   Baker WE (2000) *Achieving Success Through Social Capital*. Jossey-Bass, New York.

7   Simon HA (1977) *The New Science of Management Decision*. Prentice-Hall, Englewood Cliffs, NJ.

8   Bion W (1968) *Experiences in Groups and Other Papers*. Tavistock Publications, London.

9   Poulton BC and West MA (1993) Effective multidisciplinary teamwork in primary health care. *J Adv Nurs*. **18**: 918–25.

10   Anderson NR and West M (1994) *The Team Climate Inventory: Manual and User's Guide*. ASE Press, Windsor.

16

Project management

I ain't seen no horses run a project.
Mark Twain, *Huckleberry Finn*

In Chapter 2 (*see* p. 24), we discussed the concept of organisational culture and presented Roger Harrison's classification of organisations into 'power', 'role', 'task' and 'person' cultures. In this chapter we shall look more closely at the *task culture*, a term used to describe an organisation which revolves around projects, and consider how to get the most out of a small group when managing a task-based project. A useful general reference on this subject is a recent book by Reiss.[1]

An organisation that is focused on project work generally consists of multidisciplinary teams. Unlike a bureaucracy (which works by precedent) or a power culture (which follows a leader), the task organisation is particularly suited to dealing with challenges that have never been encountered before.

What is a project?

The simplest definition of a project is 'something which has a beginning and an end'. Some additional features of projects include the following.

- They are complex endeavours to do work which creates change.
- They have mixed objectives, especially constraints of quality, cost and time.
- They often involve people from throughout (and even beyond) the organisation.
- They are unique.

The *benefits* of project groups are as follows.

- They are transient – only existing while the problem is there to be solved.
- They recruit the skills necessary for problem resolution.
- They take decisions by consensus.
- They are not hierarchical.
- Rewards are distributed equitably among team members.

The *problems* with project groups include the following:

- uncertainty (what work will the members do when the project is ended?)
- working for two bosses (team members have a project leader and a line manager, who are often different individuals)
- conflicting work priorities (project vs. other work)
- workload (good team members are usually involved in many different projects and may therefore become overworked).

What is project management?

Project management involves the following three overlapping responsibilities:

1   ensuring that all of the project tasks are clearly defined and completed on time to the desired standard of quality
2   ensuring that the individual team members understand their role and responsibilities and are given guidance and opportunity to develop their skills
3   ensuring that the work is well co-ordinated and fairly distributed in the team to encourage effective team working.

Successful project management may be defined as achieving the correct balance between the opposing constraints of time, quality and cost (*see* Figure 16.1). The skills needed to manage a project successfully are essentially administrative, facilitative (*see* Chapter 4, p. 52), problem-solving (*see* Chapter 14)

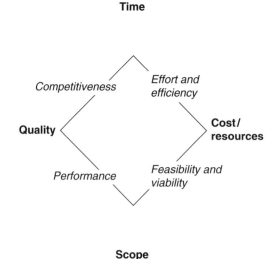

Figure 16.1:   Dimensions of project management (adapted from Turner).[2]

and leadership skills (*see* Chapter 17, p. 275). Table 16.1 summarises the steps involved in conventional project management.

Table 16.1:   Steps in project management

Step	Management process
Perceive the problem	Identify that there is an opportunity for providing benefits to the organisation
Gather data	Collect information relating to the opportunity
Define the problem	Determine the value of the opportunity and potential benefits
Generate solutions	Identify several ways of delivering the opportunity and achieving the benefits
Evaluate solutions	Determine the cost of implementing solutions, the likelihood of success and the levels of benefit
Select a solution	Choose the solution that will give the best value for money
Communicate	Tell all of the parties involved of the chosen solution
Plan implementation	Complete a detailed design of the solution, plan the implementation and freeze the design
Implement	Authorise work, assign tasks to people, undertake the work and control progress
Monitor	Monitor the results to ensure that the problem has been solved and the benefits obtained

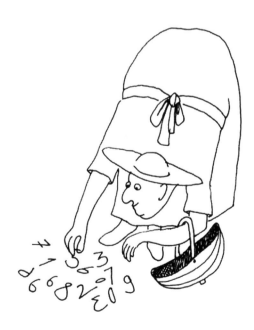

▼

Data gatherer.

An important task for the project leader is to bear in mind the four phases of the project life cycle, namely germination (proposal and initiation), growth (design and appraisal), maturity (execution and control) and death (completion, closure and evaluation). In practice these are not discrete sequential phases, because it may be necessary to redefine or re-plan at any time during the project, but they are a convenient way to introduce some discipline into the project process and ensure that certain checks are carried out at appropriate points. All of the phases are dynamic and subject to review and revision at any time.

There is often a misunderstanding about when to start a project. When everyone involved is enthusiastic about the project there is a driving need to get going, and this can lead to a disorganised and unstructured approach to the work. Success with the project is directly related to balancing the time and effort given to each of the four phases in the project life cycle. After all, a project that is beautifully planned and which develops well in the early stages is not much use if the team runs out of time or energy half-way through!

The administrative and organisational details of project management are beyond the scope of this book, but are covered in detail by other texts. In summary, the project leader must, in addition to leading his or her team, pay attention to the following:

1 managing the *scope* of the project – that is:
   • conceptualise what needs to be done and match this with the project's objectives
   • break the work down into manageable chunks
   • authorise and execute the work (ensuring that enough, but only enough, is done to meet the objectives)
   • produce, deliver or disseminate the product
2 managing the *time course* of the project via a milestone plan – that is:
   • define a time framework with intermediate products, or deliverables, which build towards the project's final objectives
   • in this plan, focus on necessary decisions and ensure that work packages are covered in the right order
   • confirm that nothing has been left out (i.e. all work is covered in the plan) and that appropriate emphasis has been given to the different areas of work
   • communicate the stages to the project team to provide structure and a common vision
   • devolve management of aspects of the project to other parties.

Some examples of project management are given in the case studies in Box 16.1.

Box 16.1:   Some examples of project management challenges

Case A

You have been asked to manage a project within your NHS Trust looking at new ways of involving staff in decision making. You have established a project steering group with a multidisciplinary membership, and this group has prepared a comprehensive project plan. Two members of the group are from the Finance Directorate and initially were high contributors to the group. However, they have been increasingly reluctant to participate in the group and now no longer make a contribution to the project at all. Although you need them to represent the finance staff and for their finance skills, you suspect that they have found that the project's aims conflict with those of the Finance Director. What would you do?

Case B

You are trying to establish a project team to develop an innovative 'shared care' scheme for children with asthma. The Trust has provided you with barely any financial resources for this project, and the senior managers, although supportive, have told you that you must identify and recruit the team members yourself. How will you identify your project team? How will you motivate them to take part in the scheme, even though they will have to continue with their existing role as well?

Case C

You have established a project team looking at developing a new approach to training and developing nursing staff. This is the first major project that you have led, and you realise that if all goes well it will provide you with a major career boost. However, two members of the project group claim to have wide experience in both project management and education, and are trying to take over. They will not listen to you and are taking the project in a direction that is not in accordance with the Trust's objectives. For example, they are proposing to spend 80% of the entire budget on a training needs questionnaire. What should you do?

Membership of project groups: Belbin's team roles

The members of a project team should be matched not only with regard to their particular skills, but also with regard to the way they will contribute to the group process and the task. Meredith Belbin identified nine important team roles which (she claimed) could be identified in advance by administering psychometric questionnaires to the individuals beforehand.[3] These roles are briefly described below.

- *The co-ordinator (or chairperson)*, as the name implies, naturally tends to chair the meetings. They are patient but commanding, generate trust, look for and know how to use ability, do not dominate proceedings, know when to pull things together, and tend to work with the talented members of the group. This person may not have a sharp intellect, but is highly committed to team goals. They are tolerant enough to listen to advice, but strong enough to reject it!
- *The implementer (or company worker)* is conservative, predictable, reliable and dutiful. They have organising ability, common sense and discipline, and are hard-working.
- *The plant* is a very creative and clever person. They have imagination, intellect and knowledge, and are serious-minded, unorthodox and individualistic. The plant can be argumentative and disregard practical details.
- *The shaper* is highly-strung, outgoing and dynamic. They are characterised by drive and a readiness to challenge inertia, complacency and self-deception. This person may have abundant nervous energy, and winning or achieving is important to them.
- *The resource investigator* is extrovert, curious, enthusiastic and communicative. They tend to explore the new and respond to challenges. This person is 'never in their office and, if they are, they are always on the telephone'. A weakness of the resource investigator is that they may tend to lose interest after enthusiasm for a new idea has waned.
- *The monitor/evaluator* is sober, unemotional and prudent. They have a high degree of judgement and discretion – perhaps even hard-headedness. This person is important at times of critical decision making because they weigh up alternatives carefully and are not swayed by emotion. Some team members may find them boring!
- *The teamworker* is socially oriented and promotes team spirit. They tend to be mild and sensitive, and have an ability to respond to people and situations. They can reduce friction within the team, minimise the wrecking tactics of difficult members and bring out the best in their fellow workers.
- *The completer/finisher* is painstaking, orderly, conscientious and anxious, with the capacity to follow through as well as being a perfectionist. This person is invaluable for 'dotting the i's and crossing the t's', but can find it difficult to delegate.
- *The specialist* is recruited for their expert knowledge or technical skills. They tend to be introverted, anxious and somewhat limited in other areas of performance and group work (the stereotypical 'anorak').

For a team to be successful, Belbin argued, the following five criteria must be fulfilled.

- The person leading the team must fit the characteristics of the chairperson and have above average mental ability.
- There must be a plant and at least one other clever member.
- There must be a good spread of team roles.
- There must be a good match between members' roles and their responsibilities in the team (e.g. if someone is a natural chairperson they should be chairing the group!).
- In the absence of particular team roles, members must adjust their contribution accordingly.

Belbin has been criticised for placing too much emphasis on selecting team members and not enough on the team's development (*see* Chapter 8).[4] There are considerable practical problems in administering a psychometric questionnaire to potential team members and then denying them membership on the basis of their 'unsuitability'! If you completed the Belbin team roles questionnaire and found that you were a 'company worker', would that make you unable to chair a group, or unable to learn to do so? Would advance knowledge that there are (for example) 'too many plants and not enough teamworkers' for the team to function effectively become a self-fulfilling prophecy?

Most organisations simply do not have the resources to construct teams on the basis of the Belbin categories. However, Belbin's categories could be discussed in a light-hearted way during the forming stage in order to raise the issue of team roles in general. Furthermore, if a 'good' team does not seem to be getting very far, it may be worth considering whether a key role is missing. For example, does the team lack a completer-finisher? Evenden and Anderson have suggested that team roles are not as immutable as Belbin implied, and that the ability to adopt different roles when the situation requires this is an important characteristic of the team player.[5]

Leading project teams

The theoretical aspects of leadership are discussed in Chapter 17 (*see* p. 272). Leading a project team can be a particularly difficult challenge. The project leader is working with and through others, using skills to energise and direct a diverse group of people to give a high performance willingly and enthusiastically throughout the project. These people come from different parts of the organisation, where every department has its own subculture that is determined at least in part by the leadership style of the departmental manager. The leader has to work with these cultural variations to create a climate of co-operation and co-ordinate the efforts of the team members without having direct line authority. The potential difficulties in this type of group are discussed further in Chapter 15 (*see* p. 252).

The autocratic leader tells people what to do, using a push approach. At the other extreme, the democratic leader encourages open sharing of information, consulting widely and asking people to do the work using a push approach. With the latter style, people may feel that their manager is asking them to 'do a favour' rather than allocate responsibility. There is no 'best' style for managing a project team, but the preferred style is contingent on the following:

- the type of work, its priority and urgency
- the way in which the team members react and behave in the environment
- the situation and the prevailing environment.

When a crisis occurs, some managers adopt a more autocratic style in the interest of obtaining a quick result. This is because it is perceived that no time exists for consultation. Therefore ideas and suggestions are not encouraged, consensus is not sought, and the actions required are dictated by command and control. The democratic style is slower, encouraging individuals to contribute their ideas and opinions, seeking a consensus in the team and motivating it to achieve results. In practice, there is often a time penalty for these processes that is not always compatible with the demands of a time-limited project.

It is important to learn to recognise which approach is appropriate at any given time in order to achieve results in the specialised situation of a project because of:

- the nature of the work, which is constrained by time and cost
- the diverse range of skills and experience of people the leader does not know well during the early stages.

It is also important to balance the three areas of project management described on p. 258 (completing the task, developing and utilising members' skills, and co-ordinating outputs). For example, a high project workload will inevitably mean limited time to support and guide individual team members. During a crisis (e.g. when approaching a deadline) there is a tendency to move into an autocratic leadership mode in order to get the action list of tasks completed. This task orientation is potentially dangerous if it is carried on after the crisis is resolved, as the team will perceive a lack of interest in teamwork or individual people. The leader should remember to step back from the current situation following any crisis and take another overview of the project.

Achieving teamwork in project groups

A successful project team consists of a carefully designed mixture of the right skills and personalities who can work together without dissension and conflict. The first time the core team comes together it must be remembered that they are a collection of individuals who may not have worked with each other before, even if they know one another. Even if they come from within the same organisation, they may be used to different subcultures and management styles. They will look to the leader to begin to establish a sense of purpose and direction. The principles of 'forming' (*see* Chapter 6) should not be overlooked. All members should know that they are in the team because they all have experience and skills that are relevant to the project. Their abilities, creativity and efforts should be harnessed to achieve a shared goal or outcome.

Maintaining motivation among the project team can sometimes be a challenge. In general, the individuals appointed to project teams are 'knowledge workers' (i.e. they are appointed for their ability to think and analyse). The work they do as part of the project team is often outside their usual line of responsibility and reward. It may not be within the project leader's power to reward their efforts financially. Instead, Turner suggests the 'five Ps' for increasing the motivation of staff in project teams:[2]

- *purpose* (ensure that the team members believe in the importance of the project)
- *proactivity* (present the project as an opportunity for members to manage their own careers, and offer the potential for them to choose their next project)
- *profit sharing* (enable individuals, through project team membership, to share in the entrepreneurial culture of the organisation)
- *progression* (membership of the project team should be seen as a learning experience which contributes to the individual's human capital)
- *professional recognition* (membership of the team can be 'put on the CV').

Defining the project

Definition is the process of turning data into something that is no longer just a wish or a hope. The definition phase is where many projects go wrong – often because there is no clear definition of the project and it has remained confused by so many different stakeholder inputs (*see* p. 267). Successful definition must involve all of the team at every step, to build their acceptance and commitment to the work of the project.

Everyone has their own ideas of what constitutes a definition, but your purpose here must be to ensure that everyone understands:

- what you intend to provide from the project
- what you do not intend to provide
- when the outcomes are to be provided
- what constraints you have identified
- what risks are involved.

For this, you will need to collect data about the needs and expectations of your customer or client, turn these needs into requirements (i.e. what you believe will satisfy the needs), derive a project definition to specify these requirements, and ask your customer or client to approve this definition. You can formalise the definition process using five essential documents as described below.

1   A project organisation chart (i.e. a listing to show who is involved in the project), recording:
    - name and job title/position
    - location
    - contact telephone/fax number and email address
    - date assigned to the project
    - name of their line manager and contact data
    - distribution list.
2   A statement of requirements derived from your discussions with the stakeholders. You must involve all the team in deciding precisely what can be provided to satisfy these needs, and this may take several meetings. The document should record:
    - the needs and expectations identified, and the individuals to whom they are attributed
    - the extent to which these needs can be met in practice
    - which needs cannot be satisfied yet, and why
    - what assumptions have been made at this stage.
3   A stakeholder list (discussed further below; *see* p. 268) to include:
    - the name of the stakeholder and their job title/position
    - their location and contact data (telephone/fax/email)
    - whether they are internal or external to your organisation
    - their ranking of importance to the project (high, medium or low).
    Date this document, because it will need to be updated as you review the list at regular intervals. Ensure that the list is distributed to all stakeholders.
4   A project objectives statement, derived from work with your customer, which records:
    - a statement of background
    - the project purpose – why are we doing this now?

- the overall project objective (in 25–30 words)
- the primary deliverables of the project with expected delivery dates
- the primary benefits to be gained, preferably quantified financially
- the cost of the project
- the skills that are required, particularly those not currently available
- possible use of subcontractors or consultants
- any identified interfaces with other active projects.

5 A scope of work statement, which includes:
- the identified project boundary limits (i.e. what you are not going to do)
- the standards and specifications that are applicable (internal and external quality standards, process specifications, customer specifications, and so on)
- sub-contract terms and conditions imposed on third parties
- any exceptions to these standards
- where the standards are kept for reference
- how success is to be measured
- any assumptions that are made.

The scope of work statement is a useful place to document any other information that supports and clarifies your project definition.

6 A risk assessment. A risk is any event that prevents the project from realising the expectations of your stakeholders. Three fundamental risks are always present:
- business risks – the viability and context of the project
- project risks – associated with the technical aspects of the work required to achieve the required outcomes
- process risks – associated with the project process, procedures, tools and techniques employed to control the project.

Beyond the project team: managing the stakeholders

All projects impinge on a range of individuals and groups beyond the project leader and the team itself. Anyone with a potential interest in the project is a *stakeholder*, and all stakeholders are likely at some stage to try to exert influence on how the project is managed. It is not possible to ignore stakeholders – they must be managed.

Perhaps the two most significant stakeholders beyond the team itself are:

- the *customer or client* – the person or group of people who expect to receive the outcomes and
- the *project sponsor* who is accountable for the project results.

However, there are many additional (and less visible) stakeholders to consider. The team members come from different departments, and their line managers have agreed to lose their resource for some of the working weeks ahead. The line managers are often *key stakeholders* – they can have a significant impact on the project if their priorities change and they either remove the team member to other duties or tell them to reduce their commitment.

All stakeholders, particularly those inside the organisation, have an agenda (which may be hidden) about what they expect from the project. It is important to clarify these expectations before the project is defined. This is not always easy if there is a political dimension to stakeholder needs and expectations – one 'need' could be to hinder or stop the project!

External stakeholders include people who expect to get an output (such as work) from the project (e.g. suppliers, contractors, consultants and possibly government departments or agencies). All have their reasons for becoming involved in the project. In many cases the project manager will have little or no authority over any of the stakeholders, and it is a formidable challenge to manage them effectively and retain their help and support throughout the project.

The stakeholders can have a significant impact on success through their direct or indirect influence on each of the areas needed to achieve the project objectives. The leader must spend much of his or her time being 'inner-directed', focusing on the project tasks, developing and maintaining good teamwork and making sure that the right skills are present in the team. However, the leader must also be 'outer-directed', spending time with external stakeholders in order to understand their needs and expectations, drawing on their skills when appropriate and keeping them informed of progress.

Identifying stakeholders is not just part of the project start-up. Many stakeholders do not appear until later in the project, so it is important to keep a look-out for new ones appearing – usually when least expected! The relative importance of each stakeholder changes with time and with the different stages of the project. If the project leader fails to recognise or co-operate with any stakeholder, they are taking a serious risk. That stakeholder could enforce views or pressurise changes to project plans at a time that is least convenient and may hinder progress.

It may be helpful to identify stakeholders as having different levels of importance for the project. The sponsor and customer are clearly of *high* importance, but others could be ranked of *medium* or *low* importance. Internal stakeholders should be informed at the outset of the strategic importance and priority of the project. This makes the job easier when they are approached later for active support of the project.

Many stakeholders have valuable knowledge and experience and, if appropriate, this should be used. Stakeholders should be brought into the project team for a time if they can make a specific contribution. However, they must understand that the day-to-day management of the project is the responsibility of the project leader, and that they must obey the rules of group membership set by the established members.

The project manager must react promptly to covert criticism or interference that erodes team spirit and promotes conflict. Poor stakeholder control can lead to chaos, confusion and demotivation of the team through their perceived interference. Important questions to address with the team include the following.

*   Who are the stakeholders?
*   Which of them are internal and which are external to the organisation?
*   What needs to be known about each stakeholder?
*   Where and how can this information be obtained?

Then gather information about each of the following aspects.

*   Can they contribute experience or knowledge?
*   What authority does the stakeholder have?
*   What exactly is their interest?
*   Why are they interested?
*   What are they expecting to gain?
*   How will the project affect them?
*   Are they in favour of the project?
*   Are there hidden agendas and, if so, what are they?
*   Are there likely to be contractual implications?
*   Will the project interfere with their operations?
*   Could they seriously hinder or block the project progress?

One way of including all of this information in an easily digestible format is to construct a stakeholder map, in the shape of a matrix or 'dartboard', with columns for the different dimensions of the project (*see* Figure 16.2).

The list of stakeholders will change or grow with time, so the project manager must draw up a list at the outset, recording the stakeholder's name, location, address (if appropriate) and contact telephone number. The stakeholder list should be distributed to all stakeholders to demonstrate that their interest is recognised. The project leader should meet with them regularly to stay updated on any changes in their needs and keep them informed of progress.

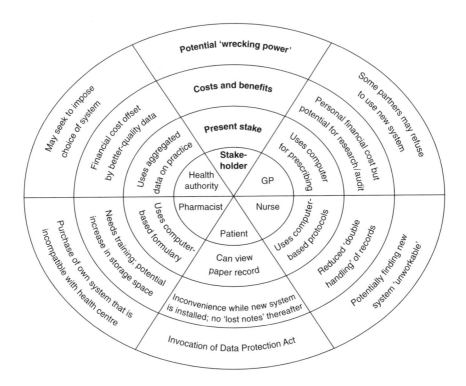

Figure 16.2: Stakeholder map drawn by a GP in a health centre who wishes to develop a 'paperless' (i.e. fully computerised) patient record system, showing the perspective of key stakeholders (fellow GPs, practice nurse, attached pharmacist, health authority and patient).

References

1 Reiss G (1992) *Project Management Demystified*. Chapman and Hall, London.

2 Turner JR (1995) *The Handbook of Project-Based Management*. McGraw-Hill, London.

3 Belbin RM (1981) *Management Teams: Why They Succeed or Fail*. Butterworth Heinemann, Oxford.

4 Clark N (1994) *Teambuilding – a Practical Guide for Trainers*. McGraw-Hill, Maidenhead.

5 Evenden R and Anderson G (1992) *Making the Most of People*. Addison-Wesley, London.

17

Leadership

> *It was a Captainish sort of day, when everybody said 'Yes, Rabbit' and 'No, Rabbit', and waited until he had told them.*
> AA Milne, *The House at Pooh Corner*

We have included this chapter in the section on small group work in organisational settings because groups tend to appoint leaders rather than (or in addition to) facilitators when they are engaged in task-oriented activities within the work environment. In other words, it is teams rather than groups (*see* Chapter 1, p. 4) that tend to seek leaders. A leader organises and directs the team's activities towards achieving a defined goal.

In practice, the role of leader is often ascribed to an individual following a discussion about who in the team might fulfil that role most effectively. A leader, especially if appointed or elected by the other team members, has both power and responsibility, and there is a substantial research literature describing studies that seek to understand the qualities of leaders and the means by which they achieve successful outcomes.

Do you have 'leadership qualities'?

First of all, remember that there is no one type of leader. Just because you do not share certain core personality traits with Margaret Thatcher does not mean that you do not have what it takes to lead a team. After all, neither did Mahatma Gandhi! Leaders do not seem to care too much about being liked – they are respected, if only for their ability to be single-minded and often ruthless. Great names behind successful corporations are seldom the people who dominate in a crowd. They work behind the scenes. As Henry Kissinger is reported to have said, leadership is often distinguished by the 'subtle accumulation of nuances, a hundred things done a little better'. Different types of leader are often divided into one of three categories, namely 'charismatic', 'inspirational' and 'transformational'.[1] Although this taxonomy has been challenged, it permeates the literature on organisational development and provides a useful starting point for considering different styles of leadership.

- *Charismatic leaders* are said to develop high levels of loyalty, identification and trust. Proponents of religious movements are typical examples of this type.
- *Inspirational leaders* 'inspire' others to set goals for themselves that, although attainable, pose challenges that require high levels of motivation and optimism. Many political leaders of western nations typify this style. It is said that followers *identify with* a charismatic leader, but *take heart from* an inspirational leader.
- *Transformational leaders* are more complex. They really act more like 'facilitators' than 'leaders' (*see* Chapter 4, p. 52), and are able to motivate people to develop themselves in new ways and to rise above their individual aims to think more widely about the needs of the group or organisation.

Gorman offers a different (but overlapping) classification of leaders into the following categories.[2]

- *The superhero leader* – aloof, thinking big thoughts, with an eye on the distant horizon. This type of leader is almost always male and enjoys a 'cult of personality' to which he generally owes his success. Superhero leaders lead from the front. Historical examples include Joan of Arc, Boadicea, Lenin, Winston Churchill and Bill Gates.
- *The democratic leader* – focused on people and staff, with a consensual and discursive management style. They seek no personal aggrandisement, but serve as a voice for the general will and a catalyst for group action. Historical examples include Gandhi and Aung San Sun Kyi of Burma (whose fight for civil rights was acknowledged by the Nobel Peace Prize in 1991).
- *The bureaucratic leader* – an expert in the organisational machine, focused on structures and systems, and using a leadership style characterised by pragmatism and attention to detail. Historical examples include Henry Kissinger and François Mitterand.
- *The reluctant leader* – achieves a leadership role by default rather than design, and given the choice would not be there at all. Once in post, they may adopt a variety of 'survival' strategies, and perhaps most commonly evolve into a democratic leader. One historical example cited by Gorman is Princess Diana. The many clinicians who find themselves in clinical director roles in the NHS would probably identify more with Brian in the film *Life of Brian* than with the late Princess of Wales!

So if you want to be a leader (or if you don't, but you find that it is part of your job description none the less), is it possible to hone your skills and, if so, how? In Chapter 4 (*see* p. 56) we showed how many of the skills of a good group facilitator can be learned through specific training, and the same is at least partly true of leadership. There is a school that says 'leaders are born' (i.e. that some innate individual qualities are essential for leadership positions, whatever the problem or context). However, research by psychologists suggests that personality characteristics alone are poor predictors of leadership ability, and has highlighted the importance of the relationship between the leader, the task content and group members.[1] Yet it is certainly true that some 'traits' characterise virtually all successful leaders – they do indeed talk more, are more motivated by success and affiliation, take a long-term view of goals (personal and organisational) and are prepared to be highly flexible with regard to how the proposed outcomes are achieved.[3] In other words, perhaps certain inborn (or acquired) traits are necessary but not sufficient for effective leadership.

Research has also shown, at least in relation to the cultural groups studied, that men are more likely to lead task-orientated projects and women are more likely to emerge in positions of social leadership.[3] There is also some evidence of an association between political leadership positions and tall stature, and the fact that many such leaders have lost a parent at an early age, thus (it is suggested) fostering an independent self-reliance that generates the confidence to take decisions and lead teams. Box 17.1 outlines the link between productivity and effective–inclusive leadership styles.

Box 17.1:   Early research into leadership styles[4]

Kurt Lewin conducted pioneering work in social psychology from the late 1930s onwards, particularly on decision-making and leadership styles. A refugee from totalitarianism, he was keen to demonstrate that a democratic method of leadership was superior to autocracy. His ability to test theoretical ideas is legendary. Indeed, he is attributed with the saying that 'There is nothing more practical than a good theory'.

Lewin organised an after-school model-making club for boys, and divided those who were interested into three groups. He arranged for confederates using differing leadership styles to guide the groups. One group had an 'autocratic' leader who made all of the decisions, another had a democratic leader who always worked by discussion about 'what' and 'how' and the third group was led using a totally '*laissez-faire*' style. The 'autocratic' and '*laissez-faire*' groups' agenda (i.e. their specific model-building tasks) was always set by the democratic group who met two days earlier and arrived at their decisions by consensual means. In this way both outcomes and processes were considered to be comparable.

The boys in the democratic and autocratic groups produced comparable outputs (models). Lewin found that the boys in the democratic group enjoyed the activity, whilst those in the 'autocratic' group became resentful of each other

continued overleaf

(though not of the leader) and eventually apathetic. The boys in the *laissez-faire* group were neither productive nor happy. Lewin then asked the leaders to switch their styles, and was able to demonstrate a reverse effect on productivity. He concluded that managerial style has a critical effect on group productivity. Many would say that this is a validation of the saying 'there's no such thing as bad soldiers, only bad officers'.

Many theoretical models have been described which suggest links between personality, situational requirements (e.g. need for high or low control, formal or informal relationships) and time frames.

- *Contingency theories* assume that a leader's effectiveness depends on the fit between his or her characteristics and the demands of the situation.[5]
- *Exchange theories* assume that leaders develop different types of 'exchange relationships' with followers, and give special attention to dyadic leader–follower pairings within groups.

Central to exchange theory is the view that leaders need to gain legitimacy in order to gain influence. Adopting group norms is an important prerequisite and a source of potential authority – breaking away from group norms can subsequently be seen as a positive attribute.[6] It is also worth remembering that elected leaders (in contrast to those appointed to that position by others outside the group) feel more able to take different decisions and put forward alternative opinions to their followers. Hollander called this accrual of influence 'idiosyncrasy credit', which allows leaders to direct change from a position of initial minority.[7] It is a risky strategy for leaders to take, because if failure occurs they face a stronger backlash.[6] Box 17.2 illustrates the growing trend to use psychometric testing techniques in combination with other assessments – the so-called 'trials by sherry' – to select individuals for leadership positions.

Box 17.2:   Selecting leaders

To illustrate the effect that research has had it is worth considering how the selection procedures have changed in a military organisation such as the British Army. It was traditional for officers (who gained leadership roles automatically) to buy their commissions, but even when this practice was stopped, recruitment took place from a selection of public schools, and ensured that the cohort came from a very narrow layer of society. It became obvious that this process did not provide individuals who had the necessary leadership qualities. Psychologists and psychiatrists were enlisted to help to devise new selection procedures. Candidates were screened using a variety of instruments and then

continued opposite

placed in situations where co-operation, communication and leadership skills were essential. Their interactions with the group and their reactions to stress were carefully assessed. In essence, this 'countryhouse method', as it became known, was the forerunner of the complex (and often lengthy) psychological assessment procedures that are now in vogue.

Adair has written extensively on leadership and motivating teams.[8] His work is openly based on command and control assumptions and may not suit the 'empowerment' cultures that have become more popular in recent management texts. Nevertheless, the notion that a balance has to be achieved between 'task, team and individual' is relevant to all leaders. Pay too much attention to task and you will fail to create a cohesive team. Pay too much attention to individuals and you may well have a good therapy session but fail to get the job done. Adair's approach to leadership is summarised and illustrated in Figure 17.1, which provides a matrix against which potential leaders can assess their behaviours.

In summary, there is evidence to support the view that leaders are both born and made. There are also those that challenge the romantic

	Key functions	Task	Team	Individual
Communication	Define objectives	• Clarify task • Obtain information • Identify resources and constraints	• Assemble team • Give reasons why • Define accountability	• Involve each person • Gain acceptance
	Plan and decide	• Consider options • Establish priorities • Plan time	• Consult • Encourage ideas • Agree standards	• Listen • Assess abilities • Delegate • Agree targets
	Organise	• Establish control • Make brief plan • Obtain feedback	• Structure • Answer questions • Prepare and train	• Check understanding • Counsel • Enthuse
	Control and support	• Maintain standards • Report progress • Adjust plan if necessary • Set personal example	• Co-ordinate • Maintain external co-operation • Relieve tension	• Guide and encourage • Recognise effort • Discipline
	Review	• Evaluate results against objectives • Consider action	• Recognise team's success • Learn from setbacks	• Appraise performance • Identify further training needs • Aid personal growth

Figure 17.1: Key functions of effective leadership (adapted from Adair).[8]

view of 'leadership' and argue that the concept is given too much weight as an explanatory model of organisational and group performance. They consider that groups attribute leadership positions because of necessity (leaders are required and therefore allocated), but that many of the leadership functions are in reality substituted and shouldered by so-called subordinates.[9] Further reading in this important research area is recommended.[1]

Practical implications of 'leadership' research

Task and relationship behaviours

It has become clear from the research performed within social psychology and management studies that there is no 'best' style of leadership or unique leader characteristics that should be selected and promoted. Successful leaders are those who can adapt their behaviour to meet the demands of their own unique situation, and to the specific tasks that face them.

One of the best known and most widely used style theories was developed by Robert Blake and colleagues,[10] who devised a grid which places concerns for individuals along the vertical axis and concern for production on the horizontal axis (*see* Figure 17.2). This led to the suggestion that managers could modify their styles and that leadership skills could be learned.

One of the most useful ways of analysing this relationship between task and leadership style has been developed by the Centre for Leadership Studies in California, and is entitled the Situational Leadership Model.[11,12] The section which follows is based on the research that this group has published. Two key behaviours form the basis of this model, namely task and maintenance (relationship) behaviours. These behaviours have been described in detail in Chapter 7 (*see* p. 124) and Chapter 8 (*see* p. 137). The research has shown that the extent to which a leader is required to provide direction (task orientation) or socio-emotional (relationship) support will vary according to the situation, particularly with the level of 'readiness' that is exhibited by a follower or group.

It used to be assumed that leadership styles were 'either/or' attributes, and that individuals could be placed somewhere along an axis with 'authoritarian' at one end and 'participative' at the other. However, this dichotomy is not seen within the practices of successful leaders. Researchers at the Ohio State University saw that the activities of leaders could be classified into two distinct

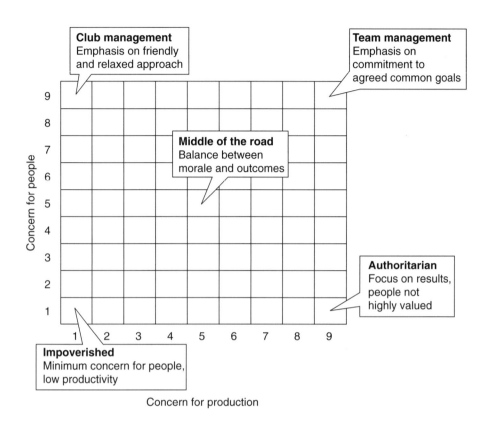

Figure 17.2: The Leadership Grid (adapted from Blake and McCanse).[10]

dimensions, namely those that initiate 'task structure' and those which consider 'relationships'. They were defined as follows:

- *task behaviour* – how much does a leader explain *to* a follower or subordinate what is to be done, by when, and exactly how the task should be completed?
- *relationship behaviour* – how much does a leader communicate *with* a follower or subordinate in order to provide emotional support and maintain social cohesiveness?

When a large group of leaders working across many different work settings was studied, no dominant style appeared. Some had high task and high relationship behaviours, others had a mixture of both, and some had low task and low relationship behaviours. The observed patterns were plotted against the axes shown in Figure 17.3. The results seemed to beg the question of which of these combinations is the most effective. Or is there another more important finding demonstrated in this data? Could it be that the effectiveness of the style depends on the context in which it is exhibited?

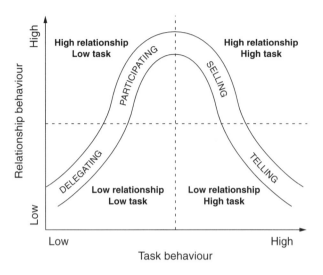

Figure 17.3:   Leadership behaviour styles.

Follower 'readiness'

The research demonstrated that there was an interaction between the behaviours exhibited by leaders and the 'willingness' and 'ability' of followers. This combination of 'willingness' and 'ability' was termed 'readiness', and clearly determined the behaviour that some (but not all) leaders chose to exhibit. This concept of 'readiness' was defined by the researchers as 'the ability and willingness of a person to take responsibility for directing their own behaviour'. The readiness was considered specific to the task that was to be performed, not as a construct of readiness at any other more general level. For example, a researcher might require a great deal of emotional and task support when asked to write a new grant application. However, neither of these may be required to complete a task that provided a high degree of intrinsic reward and in which they were extremely competent, such as proofreading a paper before final submission. For example, a secretary might be very able to transcribe a complex audiotape but the willingness to do it, compared to their willingness to learn how to use a new piece of software to publish material on the World Wide Web, might be lower. The Ohio group suggests that managerial behaviour should be carefully modified to ensure that both of these goals are achieved.

Situational leadership

The situational leadership model proposes that a leader should modify the levels of task and relationship, and that the key determinant of this flexible approach should be the readiness and ability of the subordinate (or group) to perform the specific task. As the followers' confidence and willingness increase, leaders should not only modify their task and relationship, but they also need to monitor and often reduce these behaviours in order to maximise performance. Figure 17.4 illustrates how leaders should adapt their styles according to four categories of follower behaviours. There are people who are:

- unable and unwilling to do the task – the lowest level of readiness
- unable but willing
- able but unwilling (or at least not very confident)
- able, willing and confident.

These may be simplistic classifications, but they serve as helpful rules of thumb when considering the best leadership style to use for maximum effectiveness. The important principle is illustrated by the red bell-shaped line which outlines the most appropriate leadership style for any given level of follower readiness.

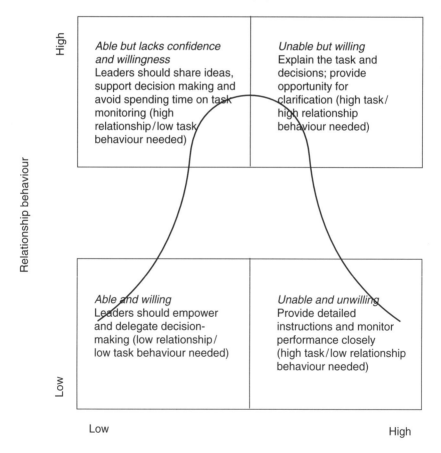

Figure 17.4

Unable and unwilling

When a group or an individual lacks both ability and willingness, a leader must define the task accurately and monitor performance closely. This is termed 'telling' behaviour, and is essentially a one-way communication whereby roles and tasks are clearly and narrowly defined. This type of leadership is often termed 'supervision', and is commonplace where work consists of routine processes, where intrinsic rewards are low, where very little training is provided or where skill levels are low. Many organisations try hard to avoid recruiting individuals who have these characteristics, but people often acquire them because of structural problems at the workplace. The effective leader's task is to motivate progression to a higher level of readiness, by increasing motivation and ability.

Unable but willing

Readiness is a not an absolute concept but a matter of degree, and the four boxes overlaid on the leadership style dimensions (*see* Figure 17.4) indicate the potential continuum that exists. Individuals can move from one area to another, and not necessarily in one direction. This model implies that leadership styles need to adapt accordingly. If an individual is unable but willing, the style advocated is one of 'selling'. The leader is still directive with regard to the task, but there is also a need to build a two-way communication process and to provide the required socio-emotional support. Followers have to be 'motivated' to buy into decisions.

Able but unwilling

People or groups in this category have the ability but lack the willingness, or at least the confidence, to perform the task effectively. The high-relationship, low-task behaviour required here is called 'participating'. It requires the leader to conduct a two-way communication in which the participants share the decision-making process and become involved in the responsibility of accomplishing the work.

Able, willing and confident

The low-task, low-relationship mode of leadership required here is known as 'delegating'. It involves accepting that the followers are 'running their own show'. It must be emphasised that introducing a high-task behaviour into this type of work group can be as disruptive as failing to provide direction in the low-ability context. The situational leadership model relies on the modification of styles and provides detailed guidance as to how and when the styles should be changed.

Modifying and adapting

This model is unashamedly based on behaviourist concepts of behaviour reinforcement, and many people will react against this analysis and the manipulative angle suggested by its proponents. Nevertheless, it is a model that has proved useful for many managers and other leaders as they grow into the roles and requirements that are expected of them.

For instance, imagine that you want to improve the 'readiness' of a subordinate who has been reluctant to take on much responsibility in the past. According to this model, a leader should be careful not to increase the level of socio-emotional support too quickly. It is suggested that the leader should provide a little less task structure whilst at the same time increasing the level of relationship behaviour – in other words, provide more 'strokes'.

Large changes would not be expected, but any movement in the desired direction should be rewarded. For example, if a leader wants a group to take on more responsibility, the leader should be less directive. If the increased responsibility leads to improved performance, it should be rewarded with an increase in supportive behaviour, praise and the offer of further consultation and participation. The model therefore promotes a two-step procedure, namely a reduction of task structure which is followed (depending on outcome) by an increase in socio-emotional support. The tasks themselves do not have less structure or purpose, but more freedom is provided for the group or for individuals to shape their work and increase the amount of intrinsic rewards generated.

It is possible to determine your own leadership style and to assess how adaptable you might be to the different levels of readiness you encounter among your colleagues. Leaders often have high scores in two separate domains. A common trend is to split between 'telling' and 'delegating', which reveals the leader who is poor at providing maintenance-type support. Another split is found between the leader who flits between 'telling' and 'participating', but who often provides these inputs at the incorrect stages. This dual effect leaves subordinates confused and it engenders mistrust and suspicion. The instrument is called the Leadership Effectiveness and Adaptability Description (LEAD). Details are available from the Center for Leadership Studies' office and website.[13]

Group and individual performance will inevitably vary over time. Crises, boredom, personal problems and other factors will inevitably prevail. A successful self-dependent work group which has tasks delegated in broad terms may suddenly become unable to perform effectively because internal conflict has occurred, and the ability to continue without any leadership support has evaporated. Similarly, an individual may be distracted by problems outside work and, although still technically able, become emotionally 'unwilling' to continue to perform effectively.

Using task-directed behaviour in such situations is an unlikely solution. However, it is all too common for leaders to have one style – be it 'telling', 'selling', 'participating' or 'delegating' – although they are unlikely to be adept leaders.

In summary, therefore, there are no universal solutions to the problem of leadership. Leaders need more than anything to learn the skills of adapting to differing group characteristics and the variation in 'readiness' that occurs at the individual level.

References

1   Bass BM (1990) *Bass and Stogdill's Handbook of Leadership: Theory, Research, and Managerial Applications* (3e). Free Press, New York.

2   Gorman P (1998) *Managing Multidisciplinary Teams in the NHS.* Kogan Page, London.

3   Eagly AH, Karau SJ and Makhijani MG (1995) Gender and the effectiveness of leaders: a meta-analysis. *Psychol Bull.* **117**: 125–45.

4   Lewin K, Lippitt R and White R (1939) Patterns of aggressive behaviour in experimentally created 'social climates'. *J Soc Psychol.* **10**: 271–99.

5   Fieldler FE (1967) *A Theory of Leadership Effectiveness.* McGraw-Hill, New York.

6   Levine JM and Moreland RL (1998) Small groups. In: *The Handbook of Social Psychology.* McGraw-Hill, Boston, MA.

7   Hollander EP (1958) Conformity, status and idiosyncrasy credit. *Psychol Rev.* **65**: 117–27.

8   Adair J (1988) *Effective Leadership.* Pan, London.

9   Calder BJ (ed) (1977) *An Attribution Theory of Leadership.* St Clair Press, Chicago.

10 Blake RR and McCanse AA (1991) *Leadership Dilemmas – Grid Solutions.* Gulf Publishing Company, Houston, TX.

11 Hersey P (1992) *The Situational Leader.* Center for Leadership Studies, Escondido, CA.

12 Hersey P and Blanchard KH (1993) *Management of Organisational Behaviour: Utilizing Human Resources.* Prentice-Hall, Englewood Cliffs, NJ.

13 Center for Leadership Studies (1993) *Leadership Effectiveness and Adaptability Description (LEAD).* Center for Leadership Studies, Escondido, CA. http://www.situational. com/

Part 5

Small groups in research

18

Focus groups

> *In my solitude I have seen things very clearly which are not true.*
> Antonio Machado, *Twenty Proverbs*

After the Second World War, an American company was disappointed and puzzled by the sales of a packet cake-mix. It had deduced (correctly) from its market research that housewives wanted the most convenient method possible to produce cakes – but why were they reluctant to buy their product? The company commissioned in-depth group interviews, and became probably one of the most well-known studies to use the method. The results revealed that the housewives felt there was something missing. For them, adding water to a powdered mixture did not equate with the sensation of 'making' a cake. Their *individual* contribution was absent, and there was a *perception* that they were not adequately involved in the process. The answer – generated by the participants through a group discussion that was gently prompted by a moderator's probing – was simple. Make the mix dependent on cracking and beating in an egg. Sales increased dramatically as a result – a significant feather in the cap of what has become known as the *focus group interview*.

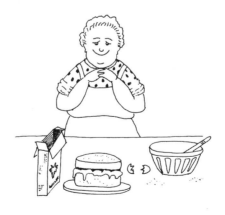

▼
The sensation of making a cake.

Origin of focus groups

It is generally agreed that focus group interviews, as a strategic interviewing method, first developed from work conducted at Columbia University in 1946. One of the professors there, Paul Lazarsfeld, was asked by the then Office of Facts and Figures (a provider of information about the war effort) to assess the public response to several radio programmes which were intended to boost morale. He took a colleague, Robert Merton, with him to the studio to demonstrate a new system he had developed. Twelve people were sitting listening to the programmes, and had coloured buttons on the sides of their chairs. Depending on their responses to the broadcast, they had been asked to press different buttons – red for positive reactions and green for negative reactions. Lazarsfeld also interviewed his groups, but Merton noticed that he used leading questions and did not allow the participants to speak for themselves. Merton was given the opportunity to 'moderate' some of the groups and the partnership flourished. The potential of the method for tapping into people's perceptions and attitudes was described in a landmark article.[1]

From those early days of gauging the effect of mass communication, the popularity of focus groups has now increased to such an extent that they are sometimes ridiculed, especially when they are used for political expediency. Between 1950 and 1980 they were seldom used outside the field of marketing research. However, once it was recognised that focus groups were able to get beneath the surface of issues, they began to be used widely in formal research studies. Survey data, although easily quantifiable, use predefined (usually closed) questions and are generally based on assumptions made by the investigator. Such surveys cannot normally discover *why* people act, think and feel as they do. Professionals in marketing and advertising wanted to look beyond numerical trends. They wanted to understand the effects of media on people's attitudes and perceived needs, but it was a difficult area to investigate. Research on group dynamics was revealing the ability of the focused interview to enable participants to voice their (often hidden) views, and to explore the basis for those opinions. A common misconception is that focus groups are only really useful for gauging reactions to products or media outputs. Arguably, the rapid uptake of the group interview by the advertising industry over the last few decades may well have reduced the credibility of the method to social scientists. A brief description of the focus group interview is provided in Box 18.1.

> **Box 18.1:** Description of the focus group interview
>
> A focus group interview is a deliberately selected cohort of individuals who are deemed to be similar (in terms of work, role or some other category) and whose attitudes and feelings about a chosen subject area are explored by a trained 'moderator'. The questions (and probes) are normally agreed before the interview, and the aim is to elicit perceptions and ideas and to uncover areas of agreement and disagreement. The proceedings are generally recorded so that transcripts can be prepared, analysed and reported. It is normal to hold several focus groups on the same subject area, to confirm conclusions until no new findings are generated.

Why use focus groups?

Qualitative research is concerned with describing, understanding and explaining, if possible, the 'nature of reality', recognising that perceptions are fundamental to our grasp of the world around us, and that therefore inevitably multiple realities exist. Quantitative data can provide information about trends and patterns, but can often fail to explain why things happen in the way they do. Knodel, for example, wanted to know more about the relationship between family size and the provision of educational support – essentially who in the family network was prepared to finance the cost of schooling. He conducted extensive surveys and the data are presented in Table 18.1.[2]

Table 18.1: Percentage of children in small and large families whose education was partially supported by sources other than parents (adapted from Morgan)[3]

	Small families	Large families
Children who lived for at least 1 year with someone other than their parents before reaching the age of 12 years	5	2
Children who received educational support from someone other than parents or siblings	5	3
Children over the age of 12 years who helped to pay their own educational expenses	8	12
Children over the age of 12 years who paid more than 500 Baht (US$20) towards their educational expenses	4	3
Children over the age of 12 years who provided support for sibling's education	8	14

However, this data is 'flat' – it reveals no understanding of the context or motives that lay behind the decisions to support educational activities. Focus group findings helped to enrich this work and, when they were combined with the quantitative data, Knodel concluded emphatically that regardless of family size it is the parents (and the parents alone) in the rural Thai settings that he studied who are expected to shoulder the burden of schooling costs. A quote from one of the focus groups illustrates a dominant theme that was elicited:[4]

> *One grandma has a lot of grandchildren. If she supports one, the others complain. The solution is to support none at all.*

> (Focus group participant)

Although data about these 'soft' issues can be obtained by techniques such as participant observation (in which researchers take part in the activities they are investigating), narrative analysis (compiling and comparing participant accounts) and ethnography (extended contact with a given community), individual interviews are one of the most widely used methods in qualitative research. So why use group interviews? What are the advantages of putting similar people together and interviewing them simultaneously?

Several important *processes* occur in groups that add to the power of the technique to uncover emotions and views that are a candid (and therefore valid) expression of a true range of opinions (*see* Table 18.2).[5]

Table 18.2:   Processes that make focus groups a useful research method

Synergy	A group interaction enables the participants to get into the subject area with more energy and enthusiasm than is often the case in solo interviews
Stimulation	Discussion generates debate, emotional reactions, counter-examples and opportunities to express solidarity of viewpoints. New ways of expressing opinions are found
Accumulation	One person's comments often generate the 'yes, I agree with that, and also...' type of statement. Interactions like this often spread and accumulate around a group if the view is widely held
Safety	A group of peers often provides the degree of safety necessary for individuals to express views which are either considered risky or that are not normally expressed outside a particular group setting (e.g. risk-taking among intravenous drug users)
Spontaneity and reflection	The unstructured format typical of focus groups allows participants to choose when to contribute. Participants normally volunteer more information in groups than within structured individual interviews. The group process is also potentially forgiving. Initial thoughts and contributions can be modified, and are often adapted during the group process. The exposure to many viewpoints allows an individual to reflect and adapt his or her thoughts if necessary

Focus groups provide opportunities for investigators to have direct contact with subjects at a level of interactive depth and candour that is otherwise difficult to achieve. They bring investigators into close contact with the research area quickly, intensely and often by having to interact with key individuals in the subject area. They ensure what is best described as *authenticity* – for an example *see* Box 18.2.

Box 18.2:   Obtaining candid viewpoints

What do parents 'really' worry about when children suddenly become ill?
Using a combination of one-to-one and group interviews with parents from a disadvantaged inner-city community of preschool children, Joe Kai found that the main concerns revolved around the possibility of children developing a fever, cough and meningitis. Parents' anxieties reflected lay beliefs, their interpretation of medical knowledge, and their fears that their child might die or be permanently harmed. Kai concluded that developing a better understanding of parents' concerns may promote effective communication between health professionals and parents. Modification of parents' personal control and perceived threat using appropriate information and education that acknowledge and address their concerns may be a means of empowering parents.[6]

Researchers who have used focus groups often comment on the 'loosening effect' of the format when the technique is used successfully. If participants are relaxed, it has been noted that opinions are shared more openly, and that their responses are more candid and reflective.[3] David Morgan and Richard Kreuger are widely known for their experience in this area and for their writing on the use of focus groups.[3,5,7,8] They have found that focus groups convey distinct advantages when the following conditions exist.

Power imbalances

Obtaining a full range of views from groups of people who are at a disadvantage in society can be particularly difficult. Literacy gaps, disenfranchisement, mistrust and the lack of any previous opportunity to communicate can severely limit information flows. This can occur within organisations or society at large when other barriers such as racial prejudice influence power relationships.

Gaps between decision makers and target audiences

This is the classic situation facing advertisers, and it explains why the technique has been used so successfully in that field. For similar reasons, broadcasters and politicians have found the methods useful. Increasingly, social scientists and clinicians are finding that the views of consumers are critically important in the design of policies or service development. Educationalists use the technique to assess needs and design curricula.

Understanding complex behaviours

Why do some middle-class males indulge in football hooliganism? Why do young teenagers often seem to avoid using contraception? Focus groups may not be able to provide statistical data that apply to whole populations – other techniques will be necessary to obtain numbers and trends. However, focus groups do have the potential to access viewpoints that may not be easy to uncover in any other way. Teenagers, the elderly and people with chronic diseases are particularly slow to express their motivations, and can struggle even to identify any conscious insights – *see* the example in Box 18.3. Provided that a conducive group climate is created, the likelihood of successful exposition of motives during the process of exploring these issues increases as the 'loosening' nature of the group interaction occurs.

Box 18.3:   Denying pain and disability

The experiences of patients who suffer from sickle cell disease were explored in focus groups by comparing the experiences of those who usually manage their pain at home with those of individuals who are more frequently admitted to hospital for management of their pain. The following key findings were reported.[9]

- The chronic nature of sickle cell disorders has been insufficiently recognised, with services oriented towards the acute management of a minority of those affected.
- Experiences of pain and patterns of hospital admission for sickle cell crises may be influenced by sociocultural and psychological factors as well as disease severity.
- The experiences of patients with sickle cell disease with regard to hospital care are characterised by mistrust, stigmatisation, control and neglect.
- Individuals who usually manage their pain at home show different attitudes and strategies with regard to hospital services to those who are frequently admitted to hospital.

Testing the nature and extent of consensus

It is difficult to gauge the extent of agreement about a topic within a particular group of people by conducting individual interviews. The range of potential viewpoints cannot be ascertained from single stances, and the focus group method has distinct advantages in this area. However, the lack of disagreement in a group cannot be equated with consensus, and moderators need to be skilled at being completely explicit in soliciting differing opinions. They are most often expressed as qualifying statements such as 'Well, I agree but ...' or by phrases such as 'but there are circumstances in which things are different'. The very fact that such exchanges occur allows what at first seem to be agreements to be explored in more depth – for an example, *see* Box 18.4.

Box 18.4:   Setting priorities for healthcare choices

Do people's views about priorities in healthcare change after they have had the opportunity to discuss and consider the implications of their choices? Ten focus groups were convened. During the interviews the participants were encouraged to discuss their views and register their opinions. These views were assessed again at second interviews held a fortnight later. The key findings were as follows.[10]

- Different techniques used to obtain the public's views may give different results.
- People's views on setting priorities differ systematically when they have been given an opportunity to discuss the issues.
- People become less willing to discriminate against smokers, heavy drinkers and illegal drug users when they have had an opportunity to reflect on and discuss their views.
- If considered opinions are required, the value of surveys that do not allow time or opportunity for reflection may be in doubt.

Exploring uncharted but sensitive areas

Difficult subjects such as beliefs among professionals about euthanasia, ideas (perhaps mistaken) about HIV transmission (*see* Box 18.5), parents' concerns when they bring children with a fever to general practitioners, and views about healthcare rationing all contain emotive issues which are seldom fully understood. It is likely that undeclared but strongly held beliefs guide behaviour. Well-conducted focus groups are likely to uncover these ideas whilst maintaining a research method which is both overt and respectful of the target subjects.

Box 18.5: HIV transmission – views about precautions

The responses of gay men to the AIDS epidemic were investigated and data were collected about their HIV status, their views about the risk they faced and the precautions they were prepared to take regarding their sexual activities. The conventional research procedure (collection of signed consent forms) would not secure the level of anonymity and confidentiality necessary for such individuals to talk freely about their views and behaviours. The normal procedures were therefore modified and steps were taken to guarantee complete confidentiality.[11]

What should focus groups not be used for?

The focus group method, like other methods that rely on self-reported data, assumes that people are valuable sources of information, particularly about themselves. Research that rests on different assumptions should not use focus groups (*see* Box 18.6). In summary, the main aim of focus groups is to provide rich, in-depth data about attitudes, ideas and perceptions in order to answer a specific research question. Qualitative research often uses the phrase 'the production of thick descriptions'.

Box 18.6: Avoid using focus groups for the following reasons

- To generate a quantitative survey of public opinion
- When confidentiality is an issue (e.g. disclosure of personal details)
- When conflicts of interest can be anticipated (e.g. an employer–employee hierarchy)
- When some members are likely to have high levels of expertise or commitment (i.e. when groups lack the necessary homogeneity)
- For covert purposes (e.g. to resolve conflicts, make decisions or change attitudes)

Over-involvement or high commitment among some members of the focus group will skew the discussion. Specialists may feel the need to appear knowledgeable and defend their positions or policies, although their attitudes and behaviours outside a 'public' discussion may be different. A group that deliberately brings specialists together would be valid, and would provide an insight into their perceptions and levels of agreement. It may be rather obvious, but focus groups should not be used for other purposes, not even covertly. They are not a means to resolve conflicts, make decisions or change attitudes (*see* Box 18.6). Groups can do all of those tasks, but what sets them apart is the purpose assigned to the activity.

What is involved in conducting a focus group?

Setting aside for the moment the practical issues of funding and recruiting (i.e. getting the right group to the right place at the right time), the most important preparatory task is to define the exact research purpose of the focus group. This can be clarified by asking 'what use will be made of the information obtained?'. These goals will vary, but typically they will include the following:[8]

- understand participant's perceptions about a topic
- identify the language that the groups use in defined situations
- generate research hypotheses for further testing
- test reactions to a product, proposal or procedure
- interpret quantitative data by placing it in particular contexts
- assess needs for educational or other development initiatives.

Eliciting the required outcomes simplifies the next – and essential – step of defining the research question and then designing the focus group process accordingly, from introduction to closure. For example, it is known that services for patients with epilepsy are not well co-ordinated between doctors who work in general practice and hospitals. Suppose you are interested in knowing how patients would like to re-design the services, and you think that focus groups would be a good method for this. The first step is to define the aims as clearly as possible. For example:

> *The purpose of these focus groups is to explore the views of adults about how the care of their epilepsy could be better co-ordinated or arranged between primary and secondary care. In order to achieve this, it will also be necessary to explore patients' views and anxieties about the way that they currently receive their care.*

The questions that should guide the focus group 'moderator' should be a refinement of the research aim, but with an eagle eye kept on the use to be made of the eventual results. An elegant way of doing this is to list the information that is needed and not needed for the research. For example:

This particular study seeks to determine:
- how patients receive care for epilepsy
- patient views about the way in which they receive epilepsy care
- which aspects of their care please or concern them
- in what ways the service could improve.

The following areas are beyond the scope of this study:
- what participants think of their doctors
- what participants think about the medication they take
- what participants think about the health service in general
- what participants think is the main problem for patients with epilepsy.

By honing these lists and thinking about the group process, it is then possible to move on to the next stage and produce a moderator's guide. This is a guide which lists the tasks, key questions and probes that will help the moderator to conduct a successful focus group, which can be repeated using the same basic framework with successive groups.

The researcher need not necessarily be the moderator. There are often good arguments for excluding the researcher from the role and finding a 'content'-free facilitator (*see* p. 50). Table 18.3 provides a brief outline and notes for a typical guide.

Participants

The ability to design and recruit the correct sample is the critical step in this research method. The commonest and most serious problem is the tendency to use a convenience sample (i.e. the nearest and easiest group that matches your requirements). The characteristics of your group should be tightly defined, and any tendency for convenience to override the chosen criteria will weaken the study. Having established the criteria for participants, it is not generally necessary to use a random method of selecting individuals for the focus groups, although that process is perfectly feasible. Focus groups are normally selected using the technique of 'purposeful sampling', whereby individuals within a defined population are selected *because* they exhibit the necessary criteria.[12]

Participants in focus groups should be similar to one another (homogenous), but in reality the degree of 'sameness' often varies. There are also focus group studies where strict homogeneity only occurs within groups, and different types of groups are used to explore the same subject. For example, the behaviour of police-officers in an urban community might be explored using groups of teenagers with differing characteristics, race or gender.

Purposeful sampling is a powerful mechanism for focusing on a specific aspect of an issue. The sample is designed to be typical of a defined group rather than representative of a wide population. Patton suggested five types of sampling strategy that can be used within the overall framework of purposeful sampling (*see* Table 18.4).[12]

The age of members is not such a critical issue, although there is some evidence that interruptions decrease and that leadership within groups increases with age. Content expertise over and above the rest of the group

Table 18.3:   Outline of a typical moderator's guide

Introductions
Welcome, putting people at ease, if necessary providing everyone with name lists and badges.
'Round-robin'-type introductions may intrude into the focus group process. Consent
procedures will have been conducted in advance of the interview

Brief outline
Give a short description of the interview's purpose. One way of emphasising this is to provide
each participant with a short statement of the research aims

Explain the focus group concept
By this stage your participants should understand why they are seated together with tape-
recorders running. If not, your consent procedures have not worked correctly. However, take
this opportunity to say the salient things about the interest you have in everyone's views,
that it is essential that only one person speaks at a time, and that you are interested in open
and honest views but will act to stop personal comments. An explanation at this point that
the process is time-limited and that you will sometimes have to curtail a discussion in order to
achieve the research aims should provide you with the necessary mandate to intervene when
necessary

Starting the talk
Participants will vary tremendously in confidence levels, and it is vital to let everyone talk,
albeit briefly, about a topic that is not threatening yet which provides some insight for the
participants about each other. The moderator should probably set a precedent by determining
the style, content and amount of self-disclosure that will be helpful for the topic area

Terminology
Every subject area has its own jargon, and this is an opportunity to check that the terms you
will be using in your questions are understood by all of the participants. Similarly, if anyone
uses a term that is not well understood, let the group know that clarifications can be
legitimately requested

A gentle beginning
The climate will be set and it is now time to engage the participants, who should be relaxed
but alert. Asking an easy but relevant question should facilitate a steady stream of responses.
The use of pauses and encouragement of body language are important at this point. Avoid
asking supplementary questions. If these are really required, use short probes

Digging in
The right time to ask about certain difficult or sensitive issues will vary according to the
contributions, levels of disclosure, humour and feeling of safety generated within the group.
Good facilitation skills are needed at this stage (*see* p. 56)

Closure
When focus groups are successful, time flies and it can be difficult to pull the threads
together. Most moderators summarise the key themes and check for general agreement on
these. A call for final thoughts or reflections often helps participants to focus on their views at
the end of the interview. Allow plenty of time for this stage, as participants often modify their
views and admit that the process has allowed them to crystallise their real feelings about the
topic

Table 18.4:   Purposeful sampling strategies

Extreme cases
These are individuals who 'deviate' from the norm, but there is a need to understand their attitudes and motives (e.g. a study to investigate the factors that would perpetuate recidivist behaviour in arsonists)

Typical cases
These individuals exemplify the norm and represent the widest membership of a group of people (e.g. the views of pupils within a band of average examination grades regarding the benefits of further education)

Maximum variation cases
This is a group in which individuals demonstrate the maximum variation (e.g. secondary school teachers with the minimum and maximum annual sick-leave records)

Politics, power or sensitivity
Some individuals are powerful (or weak) within groups. Selection based on a recognised criterion will allow insight into the dynamics that may influence decision making (e.g. middle managers in organisations who have responsibilities to both their superiors and their inferiors)

Critical cases
Individuals who are pivotal to the behaviour or characteristic under scrutiny in order to establish whether what is true for them is likely be true for other similar individuals (e.g. for women in developing countries who decide to limit the number of children they bear for economical reasons, what are the important factors involved?)

members is a factor that should exclude membership. An 'expert' who displays their authority inevitably influences the group process and the opinions obtained will be skewed. However, lack of previous contact between group members is a positive attribute. People are inclined to be more truthful and to disclose more about themselves when they are in the company of strangers.[13]

A word on ethical issues

Focus groups are not like other groups where individuals willingly agree to work together. They have been specifically designed to generate data for others to consider and usually publish. Informed consent is essential, and the researchers need to have clear policies about who has access to the information, who can analyse and report the findings and, in cases where the data are particularly sensitive, the confidentiality of participants throughout and beyond the duration of the study. It is good practice from both ethical and research viewpoints to share your reports, drafts of publications, etc., with the members of your focus groups. Participants are normally interested in the way you have reported their views, and will value the feedback. It consolidates the participation and consent to report the data and, as an added bonus, it validates the findings. Further reading is recommended if you are interested in using the technique and in developing the skills of data processing and reporting.[14,15]

References

1 Merton RK and Kendall PL (1946) The focused interview. *Am J Sociol.* **51**: 541–57.

2 Knodel J, Havanon N and Sittitrai W (1990) Family size and the education of children in the context of rapid fertility decline. *Pop Dev Rev.* **16**: 31–62.

3 Morgan DL (ed) (1993) *Successful Focus Groups.* Sage, Newbury Park.

4 Knodel J, Havanon N and Pramualratana A (1984) Fertility transition in Thailand: a qualitative analysis. *Pop Dev Rev.* **10**: 297–328.

5 Kreuger R (1988) *Focus Groups: a Practical Guide for Research.* Sage, London.

6 Kai J (1996) What worries parents when their preschool children are acutely ill, and why: a qualitative study. *BMJ.* **313**: 983–6.

7 Morgan D (1988) *Focus Groups as Qualitative Research.* Sage, London.

8 Morgan DL (1998) *The Focus Group Guidebook.* Sage, Thousand Oaks, CA.

9 Maxwell K, Streetly A and Bevan D (1999) Experiences of hospital care and treatment seeking for pain from sickle cell disease: qualitative study. *BMJ.* **318**: 1585–90.

10 Dolan P, Cookson R and Ferguson B (1999) Effect of deliberation on the public's views of priority setting in health care: focus group study. *BMJ.* **318**: 916–9.

11 O'Brien KJ (1993) Using focus groups to develop health surveys: an example from research on social relationships and AIDS-preventative behaviour. In: DL Morgan (ed) *Successful Focus Groups: Advancing the State of the Art.* Sage, Thousand Oaks, CA.

12 Patton MQ (1990) *Qualitative Evaluation Methods.* Sage, Newbury Park, CA.

13 Folch-Lyon E and Tost JF (1981) Conducting focus groups sessions. *Studies Fam Planning.* **12**: 443–9.

14 Miles MB and Huberman AM (1994) *Qualitative Data Analysis: an Expanded Sourcebook* (2e). Sage, Thousand Oaks, CA.

15 Crabtree BF and Miller WL (eds) (1992) *Doing Qualitative Research.* Sage, London.

19

Consensus research

> *When they had looked at it for some while, they fell to arguing. Some said 'no' and some said 'yes'.*
> JRR Tolkein, *The Hobbit*

As several other chapters in this book have shown, the group's opinion on a particular issue is rarely if ever the unanimous view of every member. Different types of group extract and represent the views of their members in different ways (*see* Table 19.1).

The two most commonly used consensus methods are the Delphi and the nominal group technique.[1,2] Both of these methods have a number of important advantages over unstructured group discussion.

- Decision making is not dominated by the articulate and confident members.
- Individuals with a strong vested interest, and those in perceived positions of power, do not have undue influence.
- Members are able, without losing face, to retract firmly stated opinions when persuasive counter-evidence has been presented.
- All members feel involved and are encouraged to participate.
- The tendency towards 'groupthink' (*see* p. 166) is avoided.
- Tacit knowledge (i.e. knowledge which a member has but is unable to articulate or quantify easily) can be represented.
- Many ideas can be represented over a short period of time.
- Threads can be non-linear (i.e. in contrast to a verbal group discussion, several ideas can be generated simultaneously without one achieving immediate dominance).
- If the process is well facilitated, definitive conclusions can often be reached.

Consensus methods are particularly useful when the decision-making process requires the interpretation of a complex, multifaceted, incomplete or conflicting body of evidence, or when there are other legitimate reasons why unanimity of opinion on a particular issue is unlikely.

Table 19.1:   Methods of achieving and expressing group opinion

Type of group	Purpose	Principle
Formal decision-making group (e.g. committee, task force, executive board) (*see* Chapter 14)	In a service context, to arrive at yes/no decisions on issues of strategy or policy	The group's decision is expressed as some kind of numerical average of the individuals' decisions, according to rules set out in a written constitution. For example: • 'policy changes require a two-thirds majority' • 'any member has the right of veto' • 'the chairman's decision is final'
Focus group (*see* Chapter 17)	In a research context, to explore the diversity of experience and opinion on a particular issue within a selected group of people who share a common feature	The facilitator uses the group process to draw out a range of views and test key statements against the reactions of both the individuals and the group
Consensus group	In a research or service context, to synthesise and summarise the extent to which a selected group of people agree or disagree with a set of predefined statements (and, in some instances, to resolve disagreement)	The consensus process is characterised by: • anonymity (i.e. individual opinions are elicited and ranked privately) • iteration (i.e. the process occurs in a number of 'rounds', allowing individuals to change their views) • feedback (i.e. individuals see the distribution of the group's response) • quantification (i.e. the summary statement expresses the overall group result plus a measure of dispersion (agreement or disagreement) of individual views)

    The disadvantages and limitations of consensus methods, which are discussed in detail below, include the following.

- They require a skilled and trained facilitator.
- They are inappropriate for routine meetings, bargaining, negotiation or co-ordination.
- The selection of appropriate and representative panel members is a critical determinant of the validity of the group's recommendations.
- They are limited by the size of the group, and can be extremely difficult to implement with larger audiences (but see below; larger groups can be split into smaller ones).
- The process can be experienced as mechanical and inflexible, especially if the facilitator fails to encourage creativity.
- Assertive personalities may still dominate the discussion.

- The process may not give a definitive answer to a question. Subsequent follow-up surveys, observations or documentary analysis may be necessary.

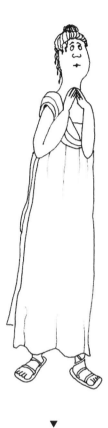

▼

Pythia: her skills of interpretation and foresight were legendary.

The Delphi technique

The Delphi technique (*see* Figure 19.1) is a structured process for collecting and distilling knowledge from a group of experts by means of a series of questionnaires interspersed with controlled feedback and discussion.

Delphi was a town on the slopes of Mount Parnassus in Ancient Greece, and the site of the celebrated oracle of the god Apollo and the earth goddess Gaea. The Delphic priests developed an elaborate ritual centred on a chief priestess called Pythia. Her skills of interpretation and foresight were legendary, and her utterances were regarded as the words of Apollo. The oracle was consulted by private citizens and public officials alike.

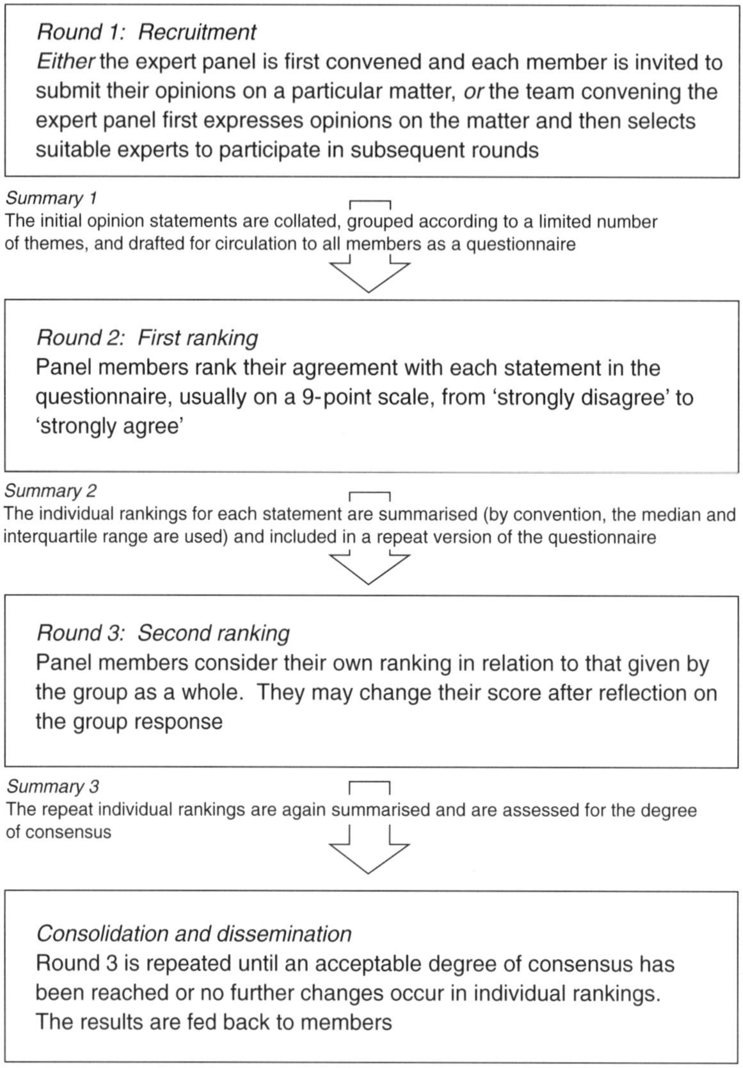

Round 1: Recruitment
Either the expert panel is first convened and each member is invited to
submit their opinions on a particular matter, or the team convening the
expert panel first expresses opinions on the matter and then selects
suitable experts to participate in subsequent rounds

Summary 1
The initial opinion statements are collated, grouped according to a limited number
of themes, and drafted for circulation to all members as a questionnaire

Round 2: First ranking
Panel members rank their agreement with each statement in the
questionnaire, usually on a 9-point scale, from 'strongly disagree' to
'strongly agree'

Summary 2
The individual rankings for each statement are summarised (by convention, the median and
interquartile range are used) and included in a repeat version of the questionnaire

Round 3: Second ranking
Panel members consider their own ranking in relation to that given by
the group as a whole. They may change their score after reflection on
the group response

Summary 3
The repeat individual rankings are again summarised and are assessed for the degree
of consensus

Consolidation and dissemination
Round 3 is repeated until an acceptable degree of consensus has
been reached or no further changes occur in individual rankings.
The results are fed back to members

Figure 19.1:   The Delphi technique.

The Delphi technique shares with this ancient tradition three important
features. First, the members of a Delphi panel are generally selected for their
wisdom and expertise in a particular topic. Secondly, the process of consulting
the experts follows a structured and prescribed format. Thirdly, the published
conclusions of a properly conducted Delphi panel rightly carry more weight
than those of a less formal decision-making process involving the same
individuals. Nevertheless, some authors object to the term 'Delphi technique'
because to them it implies a supernatural or occult influence on decision
making.

The studies that eventually led to the development of the Delphi technique began around 1944 with attempts by the US military to forecast future technological capabilities that might be of interest to them. In 1946, Project RAND (an acronym for Research and Development) was set up in the USA to study predictive methods in relation to inter-continental warfare. In 1958, two RAND researchers published a seminal paper entitled *The Epistemology of the Inexact Sciences*,[3] which argued from a philosophical viewpoint that in fields that have not yet developed to the point of having scientific laws, the testimony of experts is permissible. The problem is how to use this testimony, and specifically how to combine the testimony of a number of experts into a single useful statement.

By the early 1970s the Delphi technique had acquired academic credibility on both sides of the Atlantic, and had been formally validated and critiqued.[4] Since that time, it has been extensively used in a number of fields, particularly in healthcare and education. The RAND Corporation, in partnership with the University of California at Los Angeles, has subsequently (and somewhat controversially) applied the Delphi technique to the assessment, prioritisation and rationing of health technologies.[5] Some additional examples are shown in Table 19.2.

In the early stages of its development, the Delphi technique was used in face-to-face meetings. More recently, the technique has been used primarily via mail using self-administered postal questionnaires. Computer-based Delphi panels, administered by email questionnaires, have also been validated and are becoming increasingly popular.[6]

The Delphi technique has been both heavily promoted and extensively criticised in recent years.[1,2,7–9] There are four main issues in the ongoing debate:

- *accuracy and precision* (the extent to which the recommendations of a Delphi panel reflect the magnitude and diversity of opinion within the group)
- *reproducibility* (the extent to which another panel, composed of individuals with similar expertise, would produce the same recommendations)
- *validity* (the extent to which the group's recommendations can be trusted and relied upon)
- *usefulness* (the extent to which the group's recommendations can help in a particular area of practice).

One important determinant of both validity and reproducibility when using the Delphi technique is the professional background and level of expertise of the panel members. The Delphi method can do no more than synthesise the opinions of the group members. A group composed of individuals who are inadequately briefed on the subject matter, or who all hold vested interests, will not automatically have its inherent biases erased by three rounds of

Table 19.2:   Examples of the use of the Delphi technique

Area of interest	General format of question	Examples
Planning and policy-making	What services does a particular group of clients want and/or need? What services should we provide?[13,14]	Planning for major incidents that involve children[15] Planning an automated patient care information system that reflects the priorities of clinicians, managers and patients[16] Work-force planning[17]
Technology assessment	Do experts in the field believe that this drug, operation, educational intervention, etc., is effective and/or cost-effective?[2]	Defining generic criteria for quality assessment of randomised controlled trials when conducting a systematic review[18] Deciding which operations should be performed by day-case surgery[19]
Research	What areas of research should we focus on?[2]	Prioritisation of areas for nursing administration research,[20] paediatric research[21] and elderly care research[22]
Quality control	What is good practice? What should our performance standard be?[11]	Developing and implementing a programme for quality improvement in a healthcare organisation[23] Defining review criteria for assessing the quality of clinical management of particular medical conditions[24]
Education and training	What competencies are required for this job? What training needs to be given? What learning outcomes should this course deliver?	Identifying and evaluating characteristics of problem-based learning assignments[25] Defining appropriate tasks for pre-registration junior doctors[26] Planning curricula for nurse education[27]

questionnaires! Furthermore, 'random' variation in different panels' behaviour will inevitably lead to less than 100% concordance.

Shekelle and colleagues recently tested the reproducibility of the Delphi method in the development of criteria for defining the appropriateness of the use of certain health technologies.[10] They addressed two different health-care scenarios, namely coronary bypass grafting, and hysterectomy for non-cancerous indications. For each of these scenarios, they randomly selected panel members from an independent list of relevant professionals. Three separate panels were appointed for each of the two conditions, and their recommendations were compared quantitatively using a standard method (the three-way kappa statistic). Panel members were given a number of case scenarios describing patients with possible indications for the procedure, and were asked to rate them as appropriate or inappropriate.

Shekelle's group found that the overall level of agreement between the three panels for both coronary bypass and hysterectomy, expressed as the kappa statistic, was around 0.5 (indicating poor agreement) when assessing what constituted 'overuse' of the procedure. The proportion of procedures deemed to be 'inappropriate' varied between panels by a factor of two. However, as an accompanying editorial by Naylor points out,[11] most of the discrepancies between the panels in ths study could be explained by contextual and subjective aspects of the problem. For example, 98% of the discrepancies in the hysterectomy panel concerned indications in which pain or bleeding was interfering with the patient's daily living for more than two days per month.

Naylor claims that a high level of discordance in this particular situation should not be interpreted as discrediting the Delphi technique itself. He suggests that:

> for conditions that influence a patient's quality of life, surely the key to more appropriate utilization [of the procedure] is much greater patient involvement in decision making, not post hoc audits based on a few clinicians' judgements.[11]

In their book *Gazing into the Oracle: The Delphi Method and Its Application to Social Policy and Public Health*, Adler and Ziglio suggest that the following three key questions need to be asked before deciding whether to select or rule out the Delphi technique.[12]

- What kind of group communication process is desirable in order to explore the problem at hand?
- Who are the people with expertise on the problem and where are they located?
- What are the alternative techniques available and what results can reasonably be expected from their application?

If, as Naylor suggests, the answer to the question 'Who is the expert...?' is sometimes 'the individual patient or client in their own unique context', then the Delphi technique (or any other method of producing an abstracted and definitive summary of 'expert' opinion) will not produce results that can be consistently generalised to the individual case.

The nominal group technique

The nominal group technique (*see* Figure 19.2) is another structured group process, usually facilitated by an independent third party, which aims to identify and rank the major problems or issues of a predefined topic.[1] It is much less of a research tool than the Delphi method, and more a method of obtaining a practical result quickly. The method is effective in gaining consensus

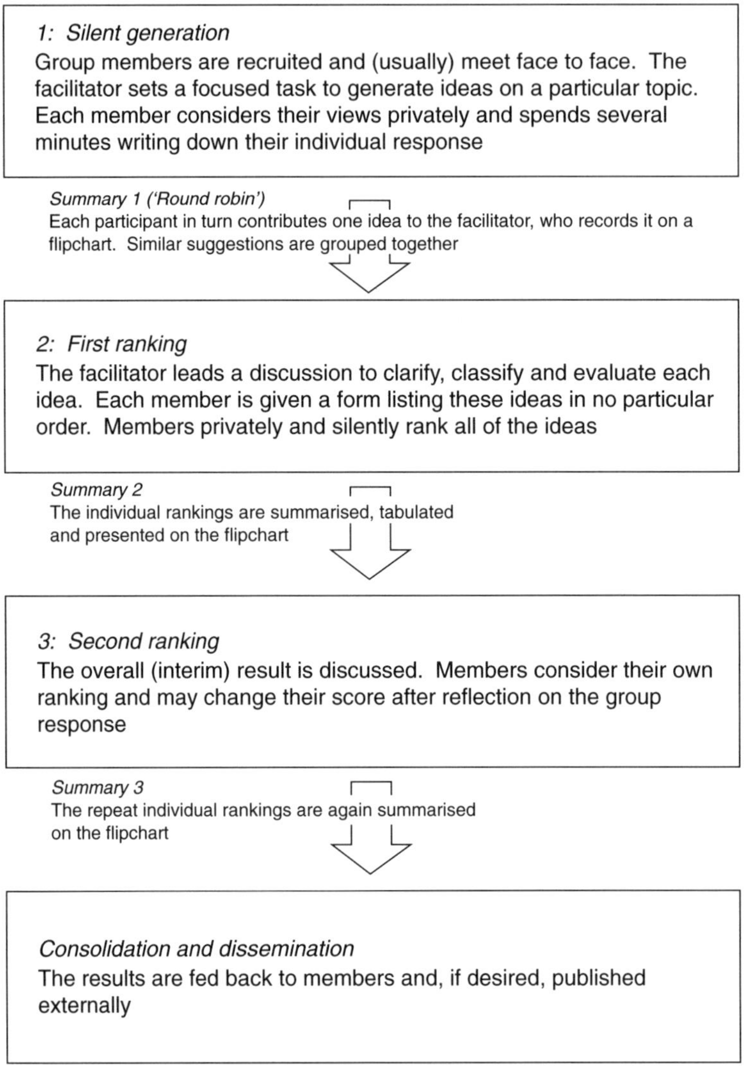

1: Silent generation
Group members are recruited and (usually) meet face to face. The facilitator sets a focused task to generate ideas on a particular topic. Each member considers their views privately and spends several minutes writing down their individual response

Summary 1 ('Round robin')
Each participant in turn contributes one idea to the facilitator, who records it on a flipchart. Similar suggestions are grouped together

2: First ranking
The facilitator leads a discussion to clarify, classify and evaluate each idea. Each member is given a form listing these ideas in no particular order. Members privately and silently rank all of the ideas

Summary 2
The individual rankings are summarised, tabulated and presented on the flipchart

3: Second ranking
The overall (interim) result is discussed. Members consider their own ranking and may change their score after reflection on the group response

Summary 3
The repeat individual rankings are again summarised on the flipchart

Consolidation and dissemination
The results are fed back to members and, if desired, published externally

Figure 19.2:   The nominal group technique.

from a wide range of types and levels of participants in a diversity of settings, especially in healthcare, social services and education. It has also been recognised as a way of generating a wide range of ideas (e.g. in situations where groups are asked to solve problems), and has been shown to be superior to brainstorming as a way of ensuring maximum participation in the process.[28] It is also used for managing participation in processes such as needs assessment, local consultation and planning, performance improvement and evaluation.

For example, a community advisory group or task force might consider using the nominal group technique at one or more of the following stages in a community development cycle:

- to determine what community problems are of immediate concern
- to decide on a more detailed assessment strategy for dealing with the identified problems
- to design improved community services or programmes
- to run a community forum or meeting where broad input is needed from lay people on a proposed plan for healthcare services, transport or education.

The nominal group technique can be completed in a single face-to-face meeting. Alternatively, the first ranking may take place by post or email and the face-to-face meeting may begin with a presentation of the first set of summary statistics. Indeed, the entire process can now be conducted via computer interaction.[29] One variation of the technique shown in Figure 19.2 that is especially useful for very large groups is for two or more nominal groups to work independently until the Summary 2 stage, and then to present their overall findings to the other groups before a third round of individual ranking. The ideal number for a face-to-face nominal group is said to be between 5 and 15 members.

The facilitator of the nominal group process should be either an expert on the topic or a credible non-expert. Recommendations for facilitating a nominal group include the following.

1   *Set-up.*
    - Start by clarifying the aim of the session and going through the process step by step.
    - Write the task down (e.g. on the flipchart or on a paper handout).
2   *Silent generation.*
    - Allow sufficient time for this phase.
    - Request all of the participants to commit themselves to paper.
    - Maintain silence.
3   *Round robin.*
    - Ask all of the participants to state the problem or issue that they feel is most important first.
    - Encourage each participant to provide at least one idea.
    - Record responses accurately – preferably on a flipchart in front of the group.
    - Give each idea a letter or number so that it can be easily identified.
    - Clarify ambiguous ideas with the person who suggested them.
4   *Discussion.*
    - Summarise what the participants have said (focusing especially on the less active members' contributions).

- Alert the group if they are wandering off the subject.
- Break down complex ideas into a number of simpler ones.
- Combine similar ideas under theme headings.
- Add new ideas if necessary.
- Delete any ideas that are considered to be irrelevant or unimportant.

5   *Ranking.*
- Generate a master list of all the problems or issues.
- Ask each member to rank the top five (or seven) problems or issues by assigning 5 (or 7) points to their most important perceived problem and 1 point to the problem considered to be least important. Issues perceived to be less important should not be ranked.
- Use postcard-sized voting cards which can be collected up and processed quickly.

6   *Summarising.*
- Tally the results by adding the points for each problem or issue. The problem or issue with the highest number of points is the most important one for the entire team.
- Discuss the results and generate a final ranked list for action planning.

Conclusion

Consensus research methods should not be dismissed as 'unscientific', but neither should they be viewed as a panacea. Used judiciously, perhaps as one of several instruments, both the Delphi method and the nominal group process can help to establish priorities, define the limits of certainty, and explore and resolve disagreement. However, sound methodology is needed to ensure the representativeness, validity and usefulness of the recommendations produced. In particular, panel members must be carefully selected, the facilitator must be competent, and the stages in the process must be strictly adhered to.

References

1   Delbecq A, Van de Ven A and Gustafson D (1986) *Group Techniques for Program Planning: A Guide to Nominal Group and Delphi Processes.* Green Briar Press, Middleton, WI.

2   Jones J and Hunter D (1995) Qualitative research: consensus methods for medical and health services research. *BMJ.* **311**: 376–80.

3   Helmer O and Rescher N (1958) *On the Epistemology of the Inexact Sciences.* The Rand Corporation, Santa Monica, CA.

4   Pill J (1971) The Delphi method: substance, context, a critique and an annotated bibliography. *Socio-Econ Plan Sci.* **5**: 57–71.

5   Brook RH, Chassin MR, Fink A, Solomon DH, Kosecoff J and Park RE (1986) A method for the detailed assessment of the appropriateness of medical technologies. *Int J Technol Assess Health Care.* **2**: 56–63.

6   Murray T and Hiltz SR (1995) Computer-based Delphi processes. In: M Adler and E Ziglio (eds) *Gazing into the Oracle: the Delphi Method and its Application to Social Policy and Public Health.* Jessica Kingsley Publishers, London.

7   Goodman CM (1987) The Delphi technique: a critique. *J Adv Nurs.* **12**: 729–34.

8   McKenna HP (1994) The Delphi technique: a worthwhile research approach for nursing? *J Adv Nurs.* **19**: 1221–5.

9   Williams PL and Webb C (1994) The Delphi technique: a methodological discussion. *J Adv Nurs.* **19**: 180–6.

10 Shekelle PG, Kahan JP, Bernstein SJ, Leape LL, Kamberg CJ and Park RE (1998) The reproducibility of a method to identify the overuse and underuse of medical procedures. *NEJM.* **338**: 1888–95.

11 Naylor CD (1998) What is appropriate care? *NEJM.* **338**: 1918–20.

12 Adler M and Ziglio E (eds) (1995) *Gazing into the Oracle: the Delphi Method and its Application to Social Policy and Public Health.* Jessica Kingsley Publishers, London.

13 Jairath N and Weinstein J (1994) The Delphi methodology (Part Two): a useful administrative approach. *Can J Nurs Adm.* **7**: 7–20.

14 Ziglio E (1996) The Delphi method and its contribution to decision-making. In: M Adler and E Ziglio (eds) *Gazing into the Oracle: the Delphi Method and its Application to Social Policy and Public Health.* Jessica Kingsley Publishers, London.

15 Carley SD, Mackway-Jones K and Donnan S (1999) Delphi study into planning for care of children in major incidents. *Arch Dis Child.* **80**: 406–9.

16 Chocholik JK, Bouchard SE, Tan JK and Ostrow DN (1999) The determination of relevant goals and criteria used to select an automated patient care information system: a Delphi approach. *J Am Med Inform Assoc.* **6**: 219–33.

17 Procter S and Hunt M (1994) Using the Delphi survey technique to develop a professional definition of nursing for analysing nursing workload. *J Adv Nurs.* **19**: 1003–14.

18 Verhagen AP, de Vet HC, de Bie RA *et al.* (1998) The Delphi list: a criteria list for quality assessment of randomized clinical trials for conducting systematic reviews developed by Delphi consensus. *J Clin Epidemiol.* **51**: 1235–41.

19 Gabbay J and Francis L (1988) How much day surgery? Delphic predictions. *BMJ.* **297**: 1249–52.

20 Lynn MR, Layman EL and Englebardt SP (1998) Nursing administration research priorities. A national Delphi study. *J Nurs Adm.* **28**: 7–11.

21 Schmidt K, Montgomery LA, Bruene D and Kenney M (1997) Determining research priorities in pediatric nursing: a Delphi study. *J Pediatr Nurs.* **12**: 201–7.

22 Ventura MR, Waligora-Serafin B and Crosby F (1989) Research priorities for the care of the veteran patient. *Mil Med.* **154**: 32–5.

23 Smith CE (1985) In pursuit of excellence via the Delphi technique. *Med Group Manag.* **32**: 44–7.

24 Campbell SM, Roland MO, Shekelle PG, Carley SD, Buetow SA and Cragg DK (1999) Development of review criteria for assessing the quality of management of stable angina, adult asthma, and non-insulin-dependent diabetes mellitus in general practice. *Qual Health Care.* **8**: 6–15.

25 Des MJ (1999) A Delphi technique to identify and evaluate criteria for construction of PBL problems. *Med Educ.* **33**: 504–8.

26 Stewart J, O'Halloran C, Harrigan P, Spencer JA, Barton JR and Singleton SJ (1999) Identifying appropriate tasks for the preregistration year: modified Delphi technique. *BMJ.* **319**: 229.

27 Mitchell MP (1998) Nursing education planning: a Delphi study. *J Nurs Educ.* **37**: 305–7.

28 Stroebe W and Diehl M (1994) Why groups are less effective than their members: on productivity losses in idea-generating groups. In: W Stroebe and M Hewstone (eds) *European Review of Social Psychology.* John Wiley & Sons, Chichester.

29 Hymes CM and Olson GM (1998) *Unblocking Brainstorming Through the Use of a Simple Group Editor.* Cognitive Science and Machine Intelligence Laboratory, Ann Arbor, University of Michigan, MI.

Index

Abilene paradox 131
academic mailing lists 203, 217–18
acceptance of group decisions 240–1
action learning sets 86–91
active participation in group work 5–7
Adair, J 275
additive inputs of individuals 29, 30
adhesive 44
adjourning *see* endings
affective integration 98
agendas
    hidden *see* hidden agendas
    project management 268
    review 131
alter ego technique 85
'ambassadors' 27
and test 140
assertive–co-operative grid 138, 139
asynchronous interaction, virtual groups
        212–13
attention-seeking behaviour 163
attention to physical environment 36
attentiveness of facilitators 55–6
audio-conferencing 205–6
audio-visual equipment 45–6
authenticity, focus groups 289
autocratic leaders 264, 273–4
'autograph' collection 100
autonomous mode of participation
        52–3, 54

'baggage', personal and professional 23–4
        dysfunctional groups 165
behaviour
    group 12, 225
    individual 12, 154–5, 162–3
    task 12, 276–8
behavioural integration 98
Belbin, RM 75, 261–3
Blake, Robert L 183–6, 276
Bligh, John 183, 184, 185
blocking 92
boardroom seating arrangement 43

'bobo doll' studies 75
body language
    dysfunctional groups 161
    facilitators 56, 69
'brains' 60
brainstorming 9, 91–2
    fishbone diagrams 234
    flipcharts 47
    reverse 92–3
Briggs, Katherine 76
buddy groups 193
bullies 60–1
bureaucracy 25
bureaucratic leaders 272
buzz groups 9, 79
    facilitation 64
    ice-breaking 109–10
    snowballing 79

cabaret seating arrangement 43
cause-and-effect (fishbone) diagrams
        233–6
chaining 98
chairperson 262, 263
chairs 41–4, 153
Challenger disaster 167–8
changing the topic 162
charismatic leaders 271, 272
charters, group 104–5
checking meaning 57
checklist technique, evaluation 152,
        156–7
circular seating arrangement 43
clarifiers 125
clocks 45
closed questions 57
clothing 37, 41, 119
coercion 240, 241
cognitive maps 36
cognitive integration 98
cognitive objectives, group techniques
        concerned with 8
cognitive tuning 130

coherence of physical environment 37
collaborations 246, 247, 248
collectivist cultures 24
comfort, physical environment 39–41
comfort zone 109
commitment
    multidisciplinary groups 244
    project management 265
    and size of group 17
committees 246, 247
communication
    leadership 275
    multidisciplinary teams 248–9
company workers 262
compensatory inputs of individuals 29
competition 161
competitive relationships within groups
        30–1
completer/finishers 262
complex teams 247
compromise 240, 241
computer-assisted learning 201–2
    see also virtual groups
concession 240, 241
conference calls 205–6
conferrers 58, 62
confidentiality
    focus groups 292, 296
    learning sets 90
conflicts 171
    resolution 137–43
    storming 116–18
confronting dimension of group activities
        53, 54
conjunctive inputs of individuals 29, 30
consensus
    acceptance of group decisions 240, 241
    focus groups 290–1
    processes, decision making 238
consensus research 299–301, 308
    Delphi technique 301–5
    nominal group technique 305–8
constructive feedback 70
context, group 21–32
    external pressures 31, 32
    formation of group 21–2
    organisational culture 24–8
    personal and professional 'baggage'
        23–4
    tasks 28–31

contingency theories, leadership 274
controlled discussion 9
conveners 254
co-operative mode of facilitation 52, 53, 54
co-operative relationships with groups 30
co-ordinators 262
coping mechanisms, environmental stress
        37
creative objectives, group techniques
        concerned with 11
creativity-in-education 217
'cringe factor', ice-breakers 105–6
critical cases 296
criticisms 171
crossover groups 80
cross-talk 143
culture
    differences 140–1
    management 250–1
    multidisciplinary groups 245, 246,
        249–51, 252
    organisational 24–8
        evaluation problems 154
        norms 121
    professional 249–51
    task 26, 27, 257
    virtual groups 208–10, 211–12
'cybercrèches' 41

Day, Christopher 35, 38
debates 59, 63
debriefing, role play 83
decision making 224, 238, 241
    acceptance of group decisions 240–1
    consensus processes 238
    devil's advocacy 239–40
    dialectic inquiry 239
    method 225
    multidisciplinary teams 244
    see also problem solving
'delegating' leadership style 280, 281
Delphi technique 299, 301–5, 308
democratic leaders 272, 273
    project management 264
depolarisation within groups 232
development
    of groups 11
        dysfunctional groups 162, 168
    of individuals 162
devil's advocacy 239–40

dialectic inquiry 239
dialogue 142
diaries, evaluation 152
difficult group members 58–68, 69
digressors 59, 62
 dysfunctional groups 162
directive facilitation 52
discretionary inputs of individuals 29–30
discussion
 controlled 9
 free 9
 guided 238
dishonesty 161, 163
disjunctive inputs of individuals 29, 30
displayed thinking 136
distance learning 201
 see also virtual groups
distancelearn-research (mailing list) 217
diversity
 conflict out of 117–18
 sensitivity to 74–7
divide and allocate 133
divisible tasks 29, 30
dominators 58, 61
 dysfunctional groups 163
Donald, Anna 180–1, 182
drinks see refreshments
dyads see pairs and triads
dysfunctional groups 159, 171–2
 causes 162–71
 identifying 160–2

echoing by facilitators 56
educational groups
 case study 191–200
 effectiveness, evidence for 175–88
 facilitating 14
 virtual groups 201–18
effectiveness of groups 15, 16
electronic whiteboards 45
Elton, Lewis 202, 215, 233
emails 203, 214
 academic mailing lists 203, 217–18
emoticons 210
emotional intelligence 75
emphasis 57
endings 93, 115
 focus groups 295
 personal feedback 94–5
 speaking rights 93–4

entertaining behaviour 163
Enthoven, A 234
enthusiasts 58, 62
environment see physical environment
environmental integration 98
environmental psychology 36
esteem needs 39, 40
ethical issues, focus groups 296–7
evaluation 147–8
 aims 147
 apprehension 92
 case study 193–8
 checklist 156–7
 coverage 148–50
 formative methods 150–1
 multidisciplinary teams 253, 255
 problems 154–6
 process reviews 152–3
 summative methods 152
evidence-based-health (mailing list) 217
evidence-based healthcare, teaching
  191–2, 199–200
 evaluation 193–8
 methods 192–3
 workshops, development 198–9
exchange theories, leadership 274
exercises 106
 imagine a map 109
 juggling 111–12
 negotiation example 108
expectation states theory 123
experience sharers 124
experiential learning 176–8
expertise 163
exploring the depths 57
external pressures on groups 31
 case study 32
 evaluation 154
extreme cases 296
extroverts 60
eye contact, facilitators 56, 69

face-to-face meetings of virtual group
  members 215
facilitation 13–15
 consensus research 300
 definition 49–50
 'difficult' group members 58–68
 dysfunctional groups 170–1
 evaluation 194–5, 197–8

feedback, giving and receiving
68–71
flipcharts 46
introductions 99
multidisciplinary teams 251–3
problem-based learning 187
resources 44
skills 54–5
stages 50–2
styles and dimensions 52–4
techniques 55–8
training 55
virtual groups 216
virtual groups 216–17
see also leadership
fast-forward technique 85, 131
feedback 150
dysfunctional groups 163–4
facilitation 68–71
learning cycle 176
observational 131, 152
feeling dimension of group activities
53, 54
fighting behaviour 163
fishbone diagrams 233–6
fish-bowl method
evaluation 152
role play 83
flight behaviour 163
flipcharts 44, 45, 46–7
focus groups 285, 300
applications 287–92
conducting 293–4
ethical issues 296–7
limitations 292–3
origins 286–7
participants 294–6
follower 'readiness' 278, 280, 281
following questions 57
follow-up stage, facilitation 51, 52
food and drink *see* refreshments
force field analysis 232–3
formal groups 4
formal multidisciplinary teams 247
formative evaluation methods 149,
150–1
forming 21–2, 97–8, 112, 115
ground rules 102–5
ice-breakers 105–12
introductions 98–101

project management 265
seats and seating 43
starting a group 98
formulating meaning 57
free discussion 9
free riding 92
Freud, Sigmund 11–12, 75
frustration 161
future basing 236, 237

games 10, 83–6, 89, 106
participation, increasing 133
problem-solving 108
survival 86, 87–8, 96
Gorman, Paul
leadership 272
mourning 93
multidisciplinary groups 243, 244,
245, 254
gp-uk 217
ground rules 102
establishing 77, 102–3
group charter 104–5
group behaviour 12, 225
group charters 104–5
group memory 135
group process 5–7
group recorders 135–6
group relations theory 11
group role of facilitation 14
groups
characteristics 246–8
definitions 3–5
groupthink 166–8, 178, 231
consensus research 299
group work
applications 16
content 5
facilitation 51–2
limitations 18
popularity 7–8
techniques 8–11
guided discussion 238
gurus 60, 61

half a vote exercise 108
Handy, Charles 25, 26, 27
Harrison, Roger 25, 141, 257
heating 40–1
Heron, J 14, 52, 53–4, 55

hidden agendas 23–4, 171
  case study 22
  dysfunctional groups 165, 166
  project management 268
hierarchical mode of facilitation 52,
    53, 54
  leading questions 57
hierarchy of needs 39–41
holding back 163
horseshoe seating arrangement 43
Human Genome Project 247
humour 62, 63, 66, 67
  see also jokers
Hunt, John 3, 11, 15, 25

ice-breakers 105–6
  examples 108–9, 111–12
  exercises, games and simulations 106–7
  'initiation rites' 110–11
  participation, increasing 133
  recurring groups with a long timespan
    78
  toys 110
  use of 107–8
  variety 109–10
ideal groups 15, 16
idiosyncrasy credit 274
imagine a map exercise 109
implementers 262
individual behaviour 12
  dysfunctional groups 162–3
  evaluation problems 154–5
individual evaluation 149
individual feedback 150
  facilitation 68–71
  observational 131, 152
individualist cultures 24
individual work 73–4
indivisible tasks 29, 30
informal groups 4
information for participants 41
information providers 125
'initiation rites' 110–11
initiators 125
inspirational leaders 271, 272
instinctive approach to problem solving
  228–9, 230
instructivist method of learning 8
interests and positions, distinguishing
  between 138–9

Internet
  academic mailing lists 203, 217–18
  virtual groups 204
interpersonal dimension, multidisciplinary
  groups 245, 246
inter-role conflict 116
interviews, evaluation 152
introductions 98–9
  focus groups 295
  methods 100
  name labels 99
  personal details, asking for 100–1
  recurring groups with a long timespan
    78
  sequenced 100
  short lifespan groups 77
  structured 99–100
  titles 101–2
introverts 60
intuitive approach to problem solving
  228–9, 230
invulnerability, groupthink 166

Jacques, D 8, 14, 152
Janis, IL 166, 167, 231
Johari window
  conflict resolution 142
  dysfunctional groups 164
  week-long groups 78
joining groups, reasons for 11–12
jokers 59, 60, 63–4
  maintenance role 124
juggling 111–12
Jung, Carl 75, 76
Justice, T 104, 110, 140
just-in-time learning 207–8

Kai, Joe 289
Knodel, J 287, 288
know-alls 59, 63
Kolb, David 176, 177

laissez-faire leaders 273, 274
leadership 13–14, 171–2, 271
  dysfunctional groups 161
  follower 'readiness' 278
  project management 260, 263–4, 268
  qualities 271–6
  situational 278–81
  and size of groups 17

task and relationship behaviours 276–8
see also facilitation
Leadership Effectiveness and Adaptability
Description (LEAD) 281
Leadership Grid 276, 277
leading questions 57
learned helplessness 75
learning
aids 110
computer-assisted 201–2
see also virtual groups
distance 201
see also virtual groups
effective 175–88
instructivist method 8
just-in-time 207–8
liberation approach 8
observational 75
problem-based (PBL) 6, 178–9, 182–8
sets 86–91
legibility of physical environment 37
Levine, JM 3, 27, 116, 144, 232
Lewin, Kurt 36, 176, 177, 232, 273–4
liberation approach to learning 8
life-lines 74
lighting 40–1
linguistic difficulties
multidisciplinary teams 248–9
virtual groups 211
lis-medical 217
lis-nursing 217
list servers 203
see also academic mailing lists
Lotus Notes 208
lurking 203–4
lying 161, 163

maintenance roles 123–5, 137
management culture 250–1
map imagining exercise 109
Maslow's hierarchy of needs 39–41
maximising tasks 29, 30
maximum variation cases 296
meaning, checking and formulating 57
meaning dimension of group activities
53, 54
memory, group 135
mindguards 166
mistrust 161
mixed relationships within groups 30

mobile phones 41
modelling 75
moderators, focus groups 287, 293, 295
monitor/evaluators 262
morality 166
motivation
dysfunctional groups 170
games 89
project management 265
mourning *see* endings
multidisciplinary groups and teams
challenges 245–6
communication 248–9
evaluating 255
facilitating 251–3
groups, teams, networks and
collaborations 246–8
'professional' vs. 'management' cultures
249–51
project management 257
reasons for 243–5
successful teamwork across
organisational boundaries 254–5
Myers, Isabel Briggs 75, 76
Myers-Briggs Type Indicator 76–7, 132

name labels 97, 99
needs hierarchy of 39–41
negotiation exercise 108
network-association teams 247
networks, characteristics 246, 248
neurotics 59, 60, 67
niches, group 17
'no cross-talk' rule 143
noise
group members 163
physical environment 41
nominal groups 93, 238, 299, 305–8
non-directive facilitation 52
non-verbal cues, virtual substitutes 210
norming 115, 119–22, 125
cognitive tuning 130
group structure and status systems
122–3
maintenance and task roles 123–5

objectives 171
dysfunctional groups 170
evaluation 149, 194
project management 266–7

observational feedback
    evaluation 152
    process consultation 131
observational learning 75
open questions 57
optimising tasks 29
organisations
    culture 24–8
        evaluation problems 154
        norms 121
    evaluation 149
    leadership 271–81
    multidisciplinary groups 243–55
    problem solving and decision making
        223–41
    project management 257–70
overhead projectors 45–6
Øvretveit, J 17, 243, 247, 248

paired exchanges 100
pairs and triads
    dysfunctional groups 163
    storming 115–16
    see also buzz groups
paper, flipchart 44, 45
paper tubes game 108
Pareto principle 236
participating styles of leadership 280, 281
participation
    active 5–7
    encouraging 133–4
    games 89
    hill 134–5
    invitation 134
    and size of group 17
passive aggressors 59, 65
pass-round questionnaires 152
pause technique 85
Pendleton feedback rules 68
perception of physical environment 36
performing 115, 129–30
    conflict resolution 137–41
    memory, group 135
    participation 133–5
    performance reviews 131, 133
    process consultation 130–2
    productivity and performance 143–5
    recorder, group 135–6

reverse argument positions 141–3
    storyboard 136
    task and maintenance behaviours 137
personal 'baggage' 23–4
    dysfunctional groups 165
personal feedback 94–5
personality 59–61
    assessment 73–7
    dysfunctional groups 165–6
person culture 26, 27
persuasive arguments theory 232
physical environment
    comfort 39–41
    flipcharts 46–7
    home vs. away 37–9
    importance 35–7
    information for participants 41
    resources 44–6
    seats and seating 41–4
physiological needs 39, 40
planning dimensions of group activities
    53, 54
plants 262, 263
polarisation within groups 232
politicians 59, 60, 66–7
portfolio support group 120
positions and interests, distinguishing
    between 138–9
power culture 25, 27
preferences, physical environment 36–7
preparatory work, facilitation 51
pressure
    external *see* external pressures on groups
    groupthink 166
Pritchard, James 243, 245, 255
Pritchard, Peter 243, 245, 255
problem-based learning (PBL) 6, 178–9,
    182–8
problem solving 223–4, 236–8
    effectiveness of groups 231–2
    game 108
    group behaviour 225
    rational vs. instinctive approaches 230
    sequence 225
    'tame' and 'wicked' problems 225–9
    task 224–5
    techniques 232–6
    see also decision making

process consultation 130–2
process evaluation 149, 152–3
process loss 143–4
process observers 124
production blocking 92
productivity 143–5
professional 'baggage' 23–4
    dysfunctional groups 165
professional culture 249–51
project groups 6
projection 131
project management 257
    case studies 261
    definitions 257–60, 265–7
    leadership 263–4
    stakeholder management 267–70
    team roles 261–3
    teamwork 265
project objectives statements 266–7
project organisation charts 266
projects
    definition 257–8, 265–7
    life cycle 260
psychodrama *see* role play
psychology, environmental 36
psychometric testing, leaders 274–5
purposeful sampling 294, 296
put-downs 163
pyramiding 79

quality circles 145
quality-management (mailing list) 217
questioners 125
questionnaires 152, 156–7
questions 57, 71

rank-pullers 59, 66
rational approach to problem solving
    230
rationale, groupthink 166
'readiness', follower 278, 280, 281
receptiveness 89
reconstruction 131
recording the group process 135–6
    virtual groups 214–15
recruitment to groups
    Delphi technique 302
    dysfunctional groups 169
    focus groups 294
    see also selection

recurring groups with a long timespan
    78–9
Reddy, BW 130, 131
reference groups 98
reflection in group work 7
    virtual groups 212
refreshments
    comfort 39–40
    ice-breaking 110
    introductions 100
rehearsing names 100
relationship behaviour, leadership 276–8
reluctant groups 22
reluctant leaders 272
replay technique 85
reporting back technique 152
research groups
    consensus research 299–308
    focus groups 285–97
    physical environment 38–9
resource investigators 262
resources 44–6, 172
    adhesive 44
    audio-visual equipment 45–6
    clock and timer 45
    culture, organisational 27
    evaluation 149
    flipchart paper 45
    multidisciplinary teams 252, 253
    optional extras 46
    'Post-it' notes 44–5
    thick-tipped pens 45
responsibility 89
reticent members 59, 64–5
reverse arguments 141–3
reverse brainstorming 92–3
reward systems 170
risk assessment, project management 267
risky shift process 231
Rittel, Horst 226
Rogers, Carl 52
role ambiguity 117
role assignment 116
role culture 25, 26–7
role innovation 117
role negotiation 141–2
role play 10, 81–3, 84–5
role reversal 85
role rotation 85
role strain 116

role transition 117
rote learning 175–6
row arrangement of seating 43

Sackett, David 192
safety needs 39, 40
Salmon, G 207, 209, 210, 215, 216
satisfaction, assessment of 194
say-writing 210
Schein, E 11, 12, 130
Schon, DA 86
scope of work statements, project
          management 267
'scouts' 27
seats and seating 41–4, 153
secretiveness 161
selection
    for groups
        consensus research 300
        dysfunctional groups 169
        see also recruitment to groups
    of leaders 274–5
self-actualisation needs 39, 40
self-censorship 166
self-consciousness about group processes
          172
self-disclosure 74, 78
'selling' leadership style 279
seminar groups 6
'sentries' 27
sequenced groups 80
sequenced introductions 100
sequenced turns 133
setting *see* physical environment
shapers 262
Shekelle, P 304–5
short lifespan groups 77–8
shy members 59, 64–5
'sideshows' 193, 195–6
Simpson Desert survival game 87–8, 96
simulations 10, 106–7
    participation, increasing 133
situational leadership model 276, 278–81
size
    of groups
        consensus research 300
        seats and seating 42, 43
        virtual groups 216–17
    of organisations 26
slide projectors 45–6

snowballing 10, 79
    ice-breaking 109–10
    participation, increasing 133
social competence 144
social exclusion, unintended 24
social integration 98
social learning theory 75
social loafing 144
social needs 39, 40
social objectives, group techniques
          concerned with 11
sociograms 153
software packages 204–5, 207, 208
speaking rights 93–4
specialised group software 204–5, 207,
          208
specialists 262
specificity
    of feedback 71
    of tasks 7
square-root technique 80
stakeholders
    map of 269, 270
    project management 266, 267–70
starting a group 98
    dysfunctional groups 169–70
    see also forming
statements of requirements, project
          management 266
status systems 122–3
stereotypes 166
stimulus–response chaining theory 112
storming 115–16, 125, 130
    conflict out of diversity 117–18
    potential role conflicts 116–17
storyboards 136
stress, environmental 37
structure
    of groups 122–3
        dysfunctional groups 169
    of group work 57
    of organisations 245–6, 254
structured introductions 99–100
structuring dimension of group activities
          53, 54
sulking 163
summarisers 125
summative evaluation methods 149, 152
superhero leaders 272
supervision style of leadership 279

supporters 85, 124
suppressed emotions 163
survival games 86, 87–8, 96
synchronous interaction, virtual groups
212
syndicate groups 6

tables 43
tacit knowledge 299
talking sticks 93–4
tame problems 226–7, 230
task achievement *see* task roles
task behaviour 12, 276–8
task culture 26, 27, 257
task forces 246, 247
task orientation 254
task roles 123–5, 137
    of facilitation 14
tasks
    nature of 28–31
    problem solving 224–5
teams
    characteristics 246–8
    definition 3–4
    network-association 247
    problem solving 224
    productivity 144–5
    roles 261–3
teamworkers 262
'telling' behaviour, leaders 279, 281
territoriality 37, 38
T-group approach 251
threading, virtual groups 212–14
timekeeping
    facilitation 57, 69
    resources 45
time-out technique 58, 150–1
timers 45

timid members 59, 64–5
titles 101–2
tolerance 117
toys 110
training
    of facilitators 55
        virtual groups 216
    of group members
        dysfunctional groups 169–70
        virtual groups 207–8
    of leaders 273
transformational leaders 272
triads *see* pairs and triads
Tuckman, B 11, 115
tutorial groups 6
typical cases 296

unanimity 166
unitary tasks 29

valuing dimension of group activities 53–4
van Ments, M 82, 83, 84
Vernon, DTA 183–6
video-conferencing 205
video projectors 45–6, 151
virtual groups
    academic mailing lists 217–18
    computer-assisted learning 201–2
    research questions 215–17
    types 202–6
    uniqueness 206–15

webCT 208
week-long groups 78
whingers 59, 66
whiteboards, electronic 45
wicked problems 227–9, 230
withdrawal 163